Acquired Long QT Syndrome

Acquired Long QT Syndrome

A. John Camm, MD, FRCP, FACC, FESC, FAHA, FCGC
Marek Malik, PhD, MD, DSc, DSc (Med), FACC, FESC
Yee Guan Yap, MB, MRCP

Department of Cardiac and Vascular Sciences
St. George's Hospital Medical School
London
United Kingdom

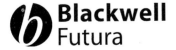
Blackwell
Futura

© 2004 by Futura, an imprint of Blackwell Publishing

Blackwell Publishing, Inc., 350 Main Street, Malden, Massachusetts 02148–5020, USA
Blackwell Publishing Ltd, 9600 Garsington Road, Oxford OX4 2DQ, UK
Blackwell Publishing Asia Pty Ltd, 550 Swanston Street, Carlton, Victoria 3053, Australia

04 05 06 07 5 4 3 2 1

ISBN: 1-4051-1838-5

Camm, A. John.
    Acquired long QT syndrome / A. John Camm, Marek Malik,Yee Guan Yap.–1st ed.
        p.; cm.
Includes bibliographical references and index.
    ISBN 1-4051-1838-5
    1. Long QT syndrome.
    [DNLM: 1. Long QT Syndrome–diagnosis. 2. Long QT Syndrome–physiopathology.
3. Pharmaceutical Preparations–adverse effects. WG 330 C184a 2004] I. Yap, Yee Guan.
II. Malik, Marek. III. Title.
    RC685.L64C35 2004
    616.1′28–dc22

                                                                            2003019461

A catalogue record for this title is available from the British Library

Acquisitions: Jacques Strauss
Production: Julie Elliott
Typesetter: Kolam Information Services Pvt. Ltd, Pondicherry, India
Printed and bound in India by Gopsons Papers Ltd, New Delhi

For further information on Blackwell Publishing, visit our website:
www.blackwellfutura.com

The publisher's policy is to use permanent paper from mills that operate a sustainable forestry policy, and which has been manufactured from pulp processed using acid-free and elementary chlorine-free practices. Furthermore, the publisher ensures that the text paper and cover board used have met acceptable environmental accreditation standards.

Notice: The indications and dosages of all drugs in this book have been recommended in the medical literature and conform to the practices of the general community. The medications described do not necessarily have specific approval by the Food and Drug Administration for use in the diseases and dosages for which they are recommended. The package insert for each drug should be consulted for use and dosage as approved by the FDA. Because standards for usage change, it is advisable to keep abreast of revised recommendations, particularly those concerning new drugs.

Contents

Preface

When he first described torsades de pointes Dessertenne did not know that there are many causes of this arrhythmia. Whilst torsades de pointes can be part of both congenital and acquired long QT syndromes, acquired long QT syndrome from pharmacological drugs is by far the most common cause of this arrhythmia. The cloning of cardiac ion channels has improved our understanding of the role of ion channels in mediating cardiac repolarization and in the pathomechanism of drug-induced long QT syndrome and TdP. As a result, increasingly more drugs have been discovered to be proarrhythmic and potentially cause sudden cardiac death. However, clinical assessment of such proarrhythmic risk is hard, if not impossible, to undertake. At times, the potential risk of proarrhythmia is often not detected during development of the compound. Frequently, the medical profession may need to rely on post-marketing surveillance and anecdotal case reports to assess the proarrhythmic risk of a new pharmacological compound, especially of a nonantiarrhythmic drug. A comprehensive literature on acquired long QT syndrome, from basic science to clinical cardiology is lacking.

This book is written with the intention of providing a detailed review on acquired long QT syndrome, from drug-induced QT prolongation to cardiac causes and noncardiac causes of QT prolongation. Detailed attention is paid to the mechanism of drug-induced QT prolongation and the clinical methodology of measuring myocardial repolarization which is crucial in the assessment of the proarrhythmic risk of a particular drug. We attempted to provide a thorough review on most of the drugs that have been reported to cause QT prolongation and/or torsades de pointes and provided our perspective towards drug-induced proarrhythmia.

The field of long QT syndrome, both congenital and acquired, is clearly advancing rapidly and they are not mutually exclusive. Indeed, whilst congenital long QT syndrome has been used as a model for explaining the proarrhythmic effects of many drugs, some patients who are carriers of the genetic mutations for congenital long QT syndrome (form-fruste of long QT syndrome) have their conditions unmasked by proarrhythmic drugs. Further insight will soon be available on the understanding of particular susceptibility to drug-induced QT prolongation and/or torsades de pointes. We hope that this book will be particularly useful for the cardiologist, electrophysiologist, pharmacologist, physician and pharmaceutical industry scientist.

CHAPTER 1

Introduction

Torsades de pointes

In 1966, Francois Dessertenne described the electrocardiographic form of polymorphic ventricular tachycardia, which he termed "torsades de pointes" (TdP) [1,2]. The word "torsades" refers to an ornamental motive imitating twisted hairs or threads as seen on classical architectural columns, and "pointes" referred to points or peaks. To further demonstrate his description, he rotated a comb along its long axis (Fig. 1.1) to show how the points of the teeth and the intermediary gap simulated the asymmetrical electrocardiographic waves of this type of tachycardia. In French, TdP means "twisting of points", and this refers to the continuously changing polarity and amplitude of the tachycardia QRS complexes. In the seminal article, Dessertenne made no attempt to suggest the mechanism of TdP and, until recently, there has been considerable conjecture as to the pathophysiology of this arrhythmia.

Since the original work by Dessertenne, it has been well recognized that many conditions may cause prolonged or abnormal repolarization (i.e., QT interval prolongation and/or abnormal T or T/U wave morphology), which is associated with TdP. Essentially, TdP may be part of either congenital or acquired long QT syndromes (LQTS). In the recent years, there is considerable renewed interest in the assessment and understanding of ventricular repolarization and TdP. There are several reasons for this. Firstly, the cloning of cardiac ion channels has improved the understanding of the role of ion channels in mediating cardiac repolarization, the pathophysiological mechanism of LQTS (congenital and acquired forms), and the pathogenesis of TdP. Secondly, there has been considerable enthusiasm for the development and use of class III antiarrhythmic drugs, which prolong repolarization and cardiac refractoriness. Unfortunately, many drugs that alter repolarization have now been recognized to increase the propensity to TdP, which is associated with syncope and can lead to ventricular fibrillation and sudden death. Finally, an increasing number of drugs, especially noncardiac drugs, have been recognized to delay cardiac repolarization and to share the ability with class III antiarrhythmics to occasionally cause TdP.

Is TdP an arrhythmia or syndrome?

Since the time of its original description, the precise definition of "torsades de pointes" has been controversial. For Dessertenne, etiological factors were not

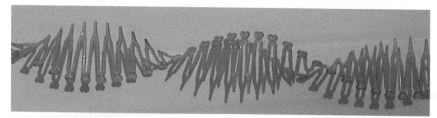

Fig. 1.1 The authors did not have a comb similar to that originally used by Dessertenne to describe TdP. However, the authors did find a circular detachable hair band that could be twisted to demonstrate how the points of the teeth and the intermediary gap simulated the pointed side and the broad side, respectively, of the asymmetrical electrocardiographic waves that formed the TdP.

an obligatory part of the definition, but rather an aid to the diagnosis. To some cardiologists, TdP is merely as an arrhythmia electrocardiographically similar to that of polymorphic ventricular tachycardia, with a set of recognized causes (congenital QT prolongation, drugs, hypokalaemia, heart block, etc.) [3]. Others described TdP as a syndrome, comprising the arrhythmia, prolonged QT interval during sinus rhythm, and a specific set of antecedent etiologies, which are included within the definition [4]. Brugada proposed that the diagnosis of TdP should require the initiation of the tachycardia by a late extrasystole [5]. Surawicz suggested that TdP is a polymorphic ventricular tachycardia associated with a prolonged QT interval or increased U wave amplitude which is amenable to suppression by an increase in heart rate [6]. El-Sherif and Turito agreed that TdP should be reserved for use in polymorphic ventricular tachycardia associated with long QT syndrome [7]. On the other hand, Coumel *et al.* mentioned that not all long QT syndrome patients with polymorphic ventricular tachycardia have a characteristic TdP configuration, and that the classic configuration of TdP can be seen without a prolonged QT interval [8]. At the end of the spectrum of views, Curtis proposed that the term TdP should be abandoned because of its confusion as to whether it represents a unique arrhythmia or clinical syndrome [9].

In practice, TdP is described as a unique form of polymorphic ventricular tachycardia that is part of a syndrome associated with QT prolongation, and usually with one or more well recognized etiological factors. In other words, it is a "chimera"—part arrhythmia and part syndrome [10]. Thus, the characteristic pattern of TdP with rapid bursts of ventricular complexes, appearing to twist around the isoelectric axis should immediately alert the clinician to the high probability of an underlying cause that should be removed or corrected, especially if it is associated with other features including QT prolongation, T wave alternans, and/or short-long-short ventricular sequence of initiation. While TdP is usually self-limiting, it may degenerate into or provoke ventricular fibrillation and sudden death (Fig. 1.2).

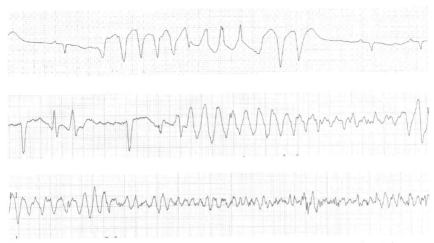

Fig. 1.2 Self-terminating TdP (top). TdP (middle) leading to ventricular fibrillation (bottom).

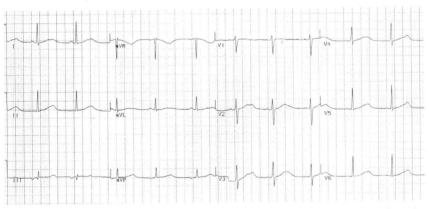

Fig. 1.3 ECG from a 24-year-old-woman who presented with TdP whilst taking cetirizine but not after discontinuation of the drug. However, the QT interval remained prolonged (QTc = 573 ms) with abnormal bifid T wave after discontinuation of cetirizine. This is probably an example of congenital long QT syndrome and the role played by cetirizine is uncertain.

Acquired QT prolongation and TdP

The congenital long QT syndromes (Fig. 1.3), which include the Jervell–Lange–Nielson syndrome (with deafness) and the Romano–Ward syndrome (without deafness), are associated with TdP and/or sudden death. The Jervell–Lange–Nielson syndrome is a recessively inherited condition whereas the Romano–Ward syndrome is an autosomal dominant condition, although there is now evidence that the inherited traits of both syndromes are not mutually exclusive. Modern molecular techniques have identified the mutations in genes encoding cardiac ion channels that cause long QT syndrome (Table 1.1), although the

Table 1.1 Genetic mutations and clinical presentations of congenital long QT syndrome.

Subtype	Chromosome locus	Gene affected	Ion channel affected	T wave	Typical clinical features
Autosomal dominant (Romano–Ward)					
LQT1	11p15.5	KVLQT1 (KCNQ1)	I_{Ks} α subunit	Broad	No QT change with exercise, syncope during physical or emotional stress
LQT2	7q35–36	HERG	I_{Kr} α subunit	Notched	Normal QT shortening with exercise
LQT3	3p21–24	SCN5A	I_{Na}	Peaked and delayed onset	Syncope during stress, rest or auditory stimuli Supra-normal QT shortening with exercise, syncope during sleep or rest
LQT4	4q25–27	Unknown	Unknown	Bizzare T wave	Severe bradycardia and atrial fibrillation
LQT5	21q22.1–22.2	MinK (KCNE1)	I_{Ks} β subunit	–	–
LQT6	21q22.1–22.1	MiRP1 (KCNE2)	I_{Kr} β subunit	–	–
LQT7	Unknown	Unknown	Unknown	–	–
Autosomal recessive (Jervell–Lange–Nielsen)					
JLN1	11p15.5	KVLQT1 (KCNQ1)	I_{Ks} α subunit	–	–
JLN2	21q22.1–22.2	MinK (KCNE1)	I_{Ks} β subunit	–	–
JLN3	Unknown	Unknown	Unknown	–	–

Table 1.2 Selected (nondrug-related) causes of acquired long QT syndrome.

Heart disease
  Coronary artery disease
  Heart failure
  Ventricular tachyarrhythmias
  Dilated cardiomyopathy
  Hypertrophic cardiomyopathy
  Left ventricular hypertrophy
  Hypertension
  Bradycardia (SA nodal dysfunction, AV block)
  Myocarditis
Metabolic abnormalities
  Hypokalemia
  Hypocalcaemia
  Hypomagnesaemia
Liver disease
  Cirrhosis
  Hepatic failure
Renal disease
Endocrine disorder
  Hypothyroidism
  Hyperparathyroidism
  Pheochromocytoma
  Hyperaldosteronism
Intracranial pathology
  Subarachnoid hemorrhage
  Cerebrovascular accident
  Head injury
  Encephalitis
Diabetes mellitus
Anorexia nervosa/starvation
Bulemia
Obesity
Liquid protein diet
Human immunodeficiency virus (HIV) infection

genetic defects in about 20% of patients are still unknown. The clinically manifested condition of congenital LQTS is rare.

The acquired form of LQTS is more common. It has many causes (Table 1.2) of which the most likely is medication. A steadily increasing number of drugs (cardiac and noncardiac) have been reported to cause QT prolongation (Fig. 1.4), TdP, ventricular arrhythmias and sudden death. Naturally, this has troubled both the drug regulatory authorities and medical communities, especially since many of these drugs do not have cardiac indications but instead are widely prescribed for self-limiting, non life-threatening disease. The risk of fatal ventricular arrhythmia is potentially large and the proarrhythmic risks of many of these drugs were not recognized until many years after they were marketed.

It is still open to speculation whether TdPs occurring due to congenital and acquired LQTS are completely separate entities. Patients with subclinical

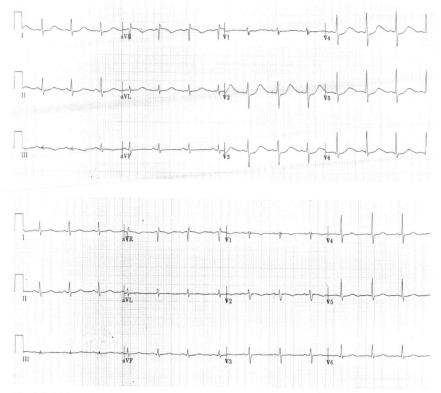

Fig. 1.4 ECGs of a 63-year-old-female patient with thioridazine-induced ventricular fibrillation cardiac arrest while in hospital. She was successfully resuscitated and this is the ECG performed immediately after the cardiac arrest (top). Note the QTc interval was 619 ms and her serum potassium level at this time was 3.3 mmol/L. The QTc interval returned to normal (399 ms) after the withdrawal of thioridazine and correction of her serum potassium level to 4.4 mmol/L (bottom). Her subsequent coronary angiogram was normal.

congenital LQTS as well as patients with non drug-related acquired LQTS are more susceptible to the development of drug-related TdP. A different degree of propensity to the initiation of TdP likely also exists between different drugs. While some drugs are likely to cause TdP in patients with relatively undisturbed repolarization, other drugs are probably capable of triggering TdP only in subjects with an underlying abnormality, e.g., subclinical congenital defect of repolarization channels.

Hence, although there are some, presumably mainly autonomic mechanisms that lead to QT interval prolongation in practically every subject (e.g., the QT interval prolongation during sleep), the pathological mechanisms and/or drugs with repolarization involvement that lead to acquired LQTS may only manifest in subjects who already have some congenital (possibly sub-clinical) abnormality of cardiac repolarization. In this sense, there is a whole spectrum of drugs and pathological stimuli differing in their propensity to cause acquired LQTS. In the drug induced LQTS, some compounds caused TdP in an appreciable number of subjects (e.g., the TdP incidence on quidine has been reported between 2.0% and 8.8% [11–14]) while other compounds cause TdP extremely rarely, only in specific subjects in whom the drug effect is combined with a highly individual repolarization abnormality (e.g., while fexofenadine is a very safe drug, it caused TdP reproducibly in a particular subject who presumably had an underlying abnormality making him particular susceptible for such a highly unusual reaction [15]). Therefore, it is not very reasonable to classify drugs into those which do and those which do not cause TdP. Rather, different drugs should be characterized by their propensity to cause the arrhythmia, ranging near zero for the very safe drugs to the induction in up to approximately 10% patients for the most repolarization active antiarrhythmic drugs.

References

1 Dessertenne F. La tachycardre ventriculaire a deux foyers opposes variables. *Arch Mal Coeur Vaiss* 1966; 59: 263–72.

2 Dessertenne F. Un chapitre nouveau d'electrocardiographie: les variations progressives de l'amplitude de l'electrocardiogramme. *Actual Cardiol Angiol Int* 1966; 15: 241–58.

3 Schamroth L., ed. 1971 *An Introduction to Electrocardiography.* Oxford: Blackwell Scientific Publications.

4 Krikler DM, Curry PV. Torsades de pointes, an atypical ventricular tachycardia. *Br Heart J* 1976; 38: 117–20.

5 Brugada P. Torsades de pointes. *Pacing Clin Electrophysiol* 1988; 11: 2246–9.

6 Surawicz B. Electrophysiological substrate of torsades de pointes: dispersion of repolarization or early afterdepolarization? *J Am Coll Cardiol* 1989; 14: 172–84.

7 El-Sherif N, Turito G. 2000. Torsades de pointes In: Zipes, DP, Jalife, J, eds. *Cardiac Electrophysiology: From Cell to Bedside.* Philadelphia: W.B. Saunders, pp. 662–73.

8 Coumel P, Leclercq JF, Lucet V. Possible mechanisms of the arrhythmias in the long QT syndrome. *Eur Heart J* 1985; 6 (Suppl. D): 115–29.

9 Curtis MJ. Torsades de pointes: arrhythmia, syndrome, or chimera? A perspective in the light of the Lambeth conventions. *Cardiovasc Drugs Ther* 1991; 5: 191–200.

10 Millar RNS. Torsades de pointes: arrhythmia, syndrome or chimera? *Cardiovasc Drugs Ther* 1991; 5: 2010–2020.

11 Selzer A, Wray HW. Quinidine syncope. Paroxysmal ventricular fibrillation occurring during treatment of chronic atrial arrhythmias. *Circulation* 1964; 30: 17–26.

12 Roden DM, Woosley RL, Primm RK. Incidence and clinical features of the quinidine-associated long QT syndrome: implications for patient care. *Am Heart J* 1986; 111: 1088–1093.

13 Kay GN, Plumb VJ, Arciniegas JG *et al.* Torsade de pointes: the long-short initiating sequence and other clinical features: observations in 32 patients. *J Am Coll Cardiol* 1983; 2: 806–817.

14 Bauman JL, Bauernfeind RA, Hoff JV *et al.* Torsades de pointes due to quinidine: observations in 31 patients. *Am Heart J* 1984; 107: 425–430.

15 Pinto YM, van Gelder IC, Heeringa M *et al.* QT lengthening and life-threatening arrhythmias associated with fexofenadine. *Lancet* 1999; 353: 980.

CHAPTER 2

Mechanisms of acquired QT prolongation and torsades de pointes

Normal ionic and molecular basis of the cardiac action potential

The cardiac action potential is generated by the changing transmembrane permeability to ion currents such as Na^+, Ca^{2+} and K^+. Like all living cells, the potential inside a myocyte cell is negative compared to the outside (resting transmembrane potential of -80 to -90 mV). However, cardiac cells are excitable and when appropriately stimulated, the ion channels within the cell membrane open and close sequentially. This changes the transmembrane ion permeability and leads to the sequential development of the transmembrane potential that is called the action potential (Fig. 2.1).

The initial depolarization (phase 0) is triggered by the rapid inward sodium (I_{Na}) and the L- and T-type calcium currents (I_{Ca-L} and I_{Ca-T}), which change the cell potential from -90 mV to $+30$ mV [1]. The transient outward I_{to} potassium

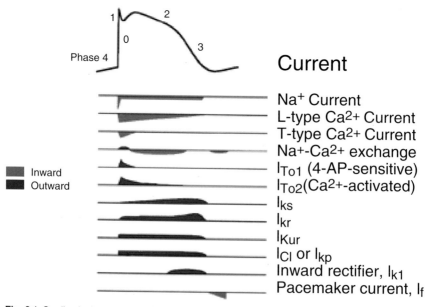

Fig. 2.1 Cardiac ionic currents and their relationship with action potential (modified from [2]).

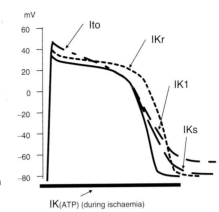

Fig. 2.2 Alteration in action potential with individual blockade of some potassium channels.

current is responsible for the slight repolarization immediately after the overshoot (phase 1). During the following plateau phase (phase 2), the cell potential is maintained by a balance between the inward L-type calcium current (I_{Ca-L}) and the electrogenic sodium–calcium exchange current (I_{NaCa}), and the outward I_{to} current. The repolarization phase (phase 3) of the myocyte is driven predominantly by outward movement of potassium ions, carried as the rapid (I_{Kr}) and slow (I_{Ks}) components of the delayed rectifier potassium current. The diastolic depolarization (phase 4) results from a combination of the decay of the outward delayed rectifier I_{Kr} and I_{Ks} currents, which maintains the resting potential at approximately $-90\,mV$, and the activation of the inward pacemaker current (I_f) and the inward sodium background leak current (I_{Na-B}). A variety of other different potassium channel subtypes are also present in the heart [2]. Pharmacological blocking and opening of each of these channels has a different effect on the action potential (Fig. 2.2).

Mechanism of acquired QT prolongation and TdP

Early after-depolarization and dispersion of ventricular repolarization

Prolongation of the action potential can be achieved by a reduction of the outward currents, particularly the outward delayed rectifier, I_{Kr} or I_{Ks} potassium currents and/or enhancement of the inward currents during phase 2 and 3 of the action potential. Among the potassium currents, I_{Kr} is most susceptible to pharmacological influence. In all presently known drug-induced acquired long QT syndrome (LQTS), the blockade of the I_{Kr} current is at least in part responsible for action potential prolongation and proarrhythmia. Blockade of I_{Kr} current results in the reduction in net outward current, a slowing of repolarization, prolongation of the action potential and clinically, QT interval prolongation and development of T- or U-wave abnormalities on the surface ECG (Fig. 2.3). The prolongation of repolarization

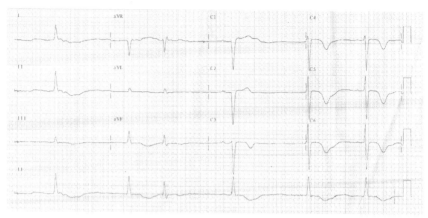

Fig. 2.3 A female patient receiving amiodarone for paroxysmal atrial fibrillation developed QT prolongation and TdP. Note the severe bradycardia and abnormal large T/U wave complex seen best in lead V1 and V6.

may result in subsequent activation of an inward depolarization current (I_{Ca-L} and I_{Na}), which generates early after-depolarizations, which in turn promote triggered activity at the end of repolarization. This occurs preferentially in the Purkinje fibers and the mid-myocardial M cell population (compared to epi- and endo-cardial cells) [3]. When accompanied by the presence of a markedly increased dispersion of repolarization, this may induce re-entry and provoke TdP, which is then sustained by further re-entry or spiral wave activity (Fig. 2.4). Thus, the presence of early after-depolarizations and dispersion of repolarization are prerequisites for the initiation and maintenance of TdP.

One reason why such activity is more readily induced in the Purkinje fibers and M cells may be related to the fact that the resting membrane potential in Purkinje fibers is more positive than that in the ventricles and the blockade of I_{Kr} channel is voltage dependent, with more block in depolarized tissue [4,5]. This may lead to dispersion of refractoriness between the two tissue types which is potentially arrhythmogenic. Similarly, compared to subendocardial or subepicardial cells, M cells show more pronounced action potential prolongation in response to I_{Kr} blockade [6]. This property results in a marked dispersion of repolarization (i.e., heterogeneous recovery of excitability), creating a zone of functional refractoriness in the midmyocardial layer, which may be the basis of the re-entry that sustains TdP.

Myocardial M cell

The term "M cell" refers to a recently described subpopulation of mid-myocardial cells with electrophysiological properties resembling those of Purkinje fibers rather than those of other myocardial cells. Differential sensitivity of M cells relative to epi- and endo-cardial cells to interventions (e.g., slowing of heart rate) or drug exposure may increase heterogeneity of repo-

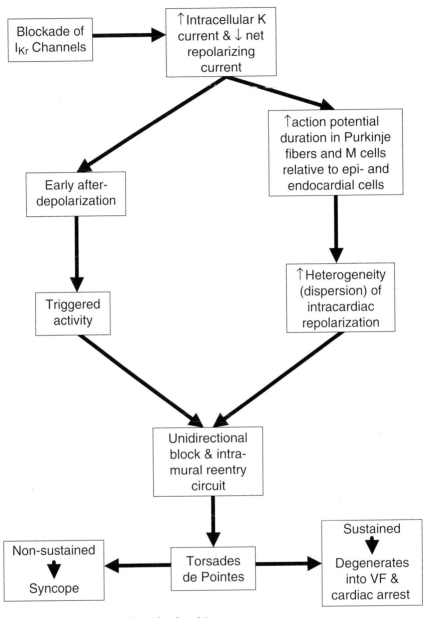

Fig. 2.4 Arrhythmogenesis of torsades de pointes.

larization across the ventricular wall (i.e., transmural dispersion of action potentials), and provide an anatomic and physiologic substrate for TdP, via transmural re-entry [3,7]. M cells have a weaker I_{Ks} potassium current and an increased late I_{Na} sodium current, both of which are believed to contribute to the long action potential duration (compared with that of epi- and endo-cardial cells) and sensitivity of the M cell to QT prolonging drugs and development of early after-depolarizations [8].

Experimental studies have shown that M cells are directly implicated in the genesis of QT prolongation and related T/U wave abnormalities, and initi-ation of TdP acquired long QT syndrome. Shimizu and Antzelevitch exam-ined the transmembrane action potential from epicardial, midmyocardial and endocardial sites simultaneously with a local transmural ECG using an arterially perfused canine left ventricular wedge preparation [9]. They have shown that the midmyocardial region is the last to repolarize and marks the end of the T wave both in normal conditions and under experimental QT prolongation (Fig. 2.5). Furthermore, induction of beat-to-beat changes in T wave amplitude and/or morphology (T wave alternans) under long QT conditions in the perfused wedge showed that this phenomenon was caused by a parallel beat-to-beat alternation of the action potential duration (repolar-ization) in the midmyocardial region, leading to an exaggeration of trans-mural dispersion of repolarization during alternate beats which will favor the

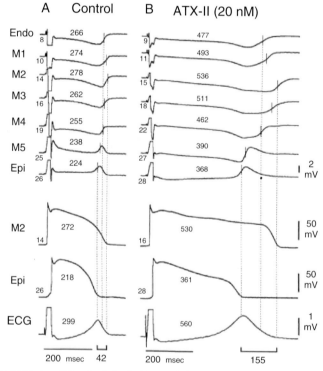

Fig. 2.5 The midmyocardial region is the last to repolarize and marks the end of the T wave both in normal conditions and under experimental QT prolongation. ATX-11, sea anemone toxin which augment the late sodium current (Ina) and produce long QT conditions similar to those caused by the defect in SCN5A, which is responsible for the congenital LQT3 syndrome (adapted from [9]).

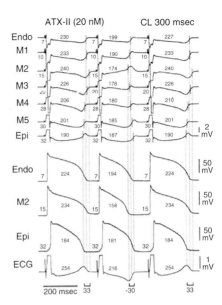

Fig. 2.6 Beat-to-beat T wave alternans under long QT conditions in the perfused wedge showed that this phenomenon was caused by a parallel beat-to-beat alternation of the action potential duration (repolarization) in the midmyocardial region, leading to an exaggeration of transmural dispersion of repolarization during alternate beats (adapted from [9]).

development of TdP (Fig. 2.6) [9]. It has thus been suggested that TdP is initiated by early after-depolarization-induced triggered activity in the M cells and is maintained by a re-entrant mechanism, created by an increase in the spatial dispersion of repolarization in the abnormal midmyocardium [10].

Short-long-short ventricular cycle

Kay *et al.* first described a characteristic short-long-short ventricular initiating sequence prior to the onset of TdP, particularly in acquired long QT syndrome (Fig. 2.7) [11]. However, the development of a postpause T- or U-wave abnormality is also seen when the arrhythmia is initiated [12]. The first ventricular complex of the sequence is generally a ventricular ectopic beat or the last beat of a salvo of ventricular premature beats. This is followed by a postectopic pause and a subsequent sinus beat. The sinus beat frequently has an exaggerated U wave. A premature ventricular beat arises from this exaggerated U wave and precipitates the onset of TdP. (Some actually speculate that this unusually large U wave is not a true U wave but a bizarre depolarization pattern due to an after-depolarization that captures a large myocardial region.) This stereotypical short-long-short cycle length changes and the presence of a postpause U wave constitute the typical pattern of initiation of TdP. This observation was subsequently confirmed by Roden *et al.* who summarized the pattern as "short cycle–long cycle–long QT–late premature ventricular complex" [13,14].

Both the abnormal T and U waves and a single ectopic impulse that follow a postectopic pause may be regarded as a warning sign of an impending TdP.

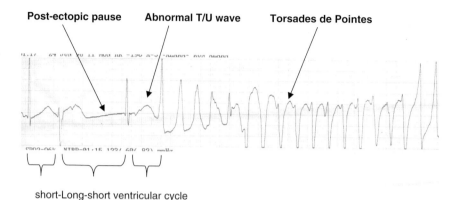

Fig. 2.7 Long-short ventricular cycle, pause-dependent QT prolongation and abnormal U wave leading to torsades de pointes.

In patients with TdP, Jackman noticed that faster prepause rates and/or longer pauses resulted in larger postpause U waves, which were more arrhythmogenic and caused faster episodes of tachycardia [15]. It is therefore important to examine the T/U wave in postventricular ectopic sinus beats, especially in patients thought to be at risk of TdP. The absence of a postpause abnormal T wave or U wave on ECG does not preclude the presence of an early after-depolarization at cellular level, since it can presumably occur in a mass of myocardium too small to produce electrical changes on the surface ECG [16]. In some patients, postpause accentuation of the U wave, if present, may be a better predictor of TdP than the duration of the QT interval, particularly with drug-associated TdP.

El-Sherif and colleagues provided an insight into the electrophysiologic changes associated with the transition of short-long-short sequence to TdP in an induced long QT condition in a canine model [17]. They observed that the short-long cardiac sequence in the form of a premature ventricular beat coupled to the long QT interval of the sinus beat commonly preceded the occurrence of ventricular tachycardia via two different electrophysiologic mechanisms. In the first mechanism, the occurrence of a second subendocardial focal activity arising from a different site to the first subendocardial focal activity, infringed on the pattern of dispersion of repolarization of the first subendocardial focal activity, resulting in multiple zones of functional conduction block and a circulating wavefront, which then initiated a re-entrant excitation [17]. In the second mechanism, a slight lengthening in one or more preceding cycle lengths resulted in prolongation of the QT interval of the sinus beat and the occurrence of a single ventricular premature beat, which was then followed, after a compensatory pause, by a sinus beat, creating the long-short sequence. The sinus beat that followed the long-short sequence showed further prolongation of the QT interval, resulting in a second ventricular premature beat of different origin, which initiated the ventricular tachycardia. In this mechanism, the authors further showed that lengthening the preceding cycle lengths produced differentially a greater degree of prolongation of repolarization at midmyocardial and endocardial sites compared with epicardial sites (cardiac memory, see below) and resulted in an increase of the spatial dispersion of repolarization. The increased dispersion of repolarization at key adjacent sites resulted in the development of *de novo* zones of functional conduction block and/or slowed conduction that created the necessary prerequisites for successful re-entry [17]. In ventricular myocardium, the refractory period is dependent on the preceding cycle length with the greatest effect from the immediately preceding cycle length, the so-called cardiac memory [18]. If the change in the preceding cycle length is maintained, several cycles will be required before a steady state of refractoriness is reached. M cells had the greater change of action potential duration with change in cycle length [3], thus significantly altering the transmural gradient for repolarization.

The TdP associated with acquired long QT syndrome is sometimes classified as pause-dependent TdP because the tachycardia generally occurs during a slow heart rate or in response to a short-long-short ventricular sequence, whereas in some congenital long QT syndromes, the TdP is classified as adrenergic-dependent because it is generally triggered by adrenergic activation or enhancement of sympathetic tone [15]. However, such distinctions are not mutually exclusive. For instance, adrenergic-dependent TdP is more likely to occur in the presence of pauses or slow heart rates. Similarly, adrenergic stimulation may facilitate drug-induced TdP [19], although the effect of β_1-stimulation on early after-depolarizations is controversial in that β_1-stimulation can both enhance and inhibit early after-depolarizations by stimulating both inward calcium current and outward delayed rectifier and I_{to} potassium currents, through phosphorylation [1,19].

The paradigm of activation pattern during TdP

While the short-long-short initiating sequence of TdP is now understood, the electrophysiologic mechanism of the periodic transition of the QRS axis during TdP is not fully explained. Since the original work by Dessertenne, the search for an understanding of the mechanism behind the twisting QRS morphology of TdP continues up to this date. Dessertenne initially speculated that the mechanism for the polymorphism of TdP probably arose from the presence of two automatic foci, competing for excitation of the ventricle, thus creating the changing morphology of QRS complexes, but he subsequently abandoned this possibility [20]. The possibility of two arrhythmic centres exiting activating waves into the ventricles at slightly different frequencies and competing for the extent of myocardium activated at each cycle may suggest a mechanism for TdP. However it can be shown both experimentally as well as theoretically, including mathematical modelling, that such a hypothesis is flawed and cannot lead to the gradual twisting of electrical axis within the TdP episode [21]. Dessertenne then postulated that it could be due to a single stable focus that had access to the ventricle through more than one exit. With this mechanism, the ventricles had a large re-entry circuit such that the conduction in the ventricles was greatly reduced with a subsequent increase in the refractory periods such that a stable re-entry circuit could not be maintained. Consequently, the re-entry pathway progressively changed, which explained the continuous changes of the electrical axis of TdP.

El-Sherif and colleagues performed a detailed analysis of the ventricular three-dimensional activation patterns and provided the first explanation of the mechanism of changing ventricular axis during TdP [22]. They conducted the studies on a surrogate canine model of the LQT3 syndrome by using the neurotoxin, anthopleurin-A. Three-dimensional isochronal maps of ventricular activation were constructed from 256 bipolar electrograms obtained from the use of 64 plunge needle electrodes. Detailed activation maps could be accurately constructed during QRS-axis transitions on the surface ECGs during TdP.

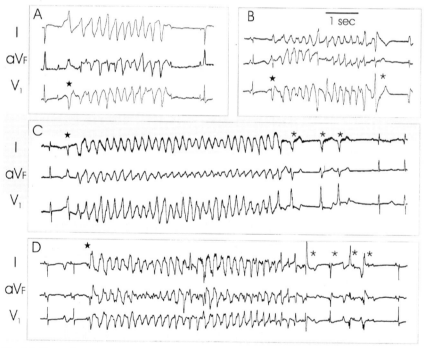

Fig. 2.8 Three-dimensional ventricular activation showed that the initiating beat of each episode of TdP arose as focal subendocardial activity (marked by stars). Subsequent beats of TdP were always due to intramural re-entrant excitation. In some episodes of TdP VT, after termination of re-entrant excitation, one or more beats of varying subendocardial focal origin (marked by asterisks) could occur at irregular and consistently longer CLs compared with CLs of re-entrant excitation (adapted from [22]).

The initial beat of all VTs consistently arose as a subendocardial focal activity, whereas subsequent beats were due to re-entrant excitation in the form of rotating scrolls (Fig. 2.8). The TdP ended when re-entrant excitation was terminated. Two different mechanisms were noted to explain this phenomenon. In the majority of TdP ventricular tachycardia, the transition in QRS axis coincided with the transient bifurcation of a predominantly single rotating scroll into two simultaneous scrolls involving both the right ventricle and left ventricle separately (Fig. 2.9). The common mechanism for initiation or termination of bifurcation was the development of functional conduction block between the anterior or posterior right ventricular free wall and the ventricular septum. In a few episodes of TdP, a fast polymorphic VT, with an apparent shift in QRS axis, was due to a predominantly single localized circuit that varied its location and orientation from beat to beat, with the majority of ventricular myocardium being activated in a centrifugal pattern.

Intrinsic factors modulating repolarization

Some evidence suggests that patients with acquired long QT syndrome have some underlying predisposition to proarrythmia. One important factor in the genesis of TdP is the particular intrinsic predisposition of an individual. For instance, it is known that most drugs that cause the development of early after-depolarizations and TdP, block the I_{Kr} channel. However, the incidence of TdP remains low and not all drugs that block I_{Kr} have the same arrhythmogenic potential. Furthermore, patients with drug-induced TdP were observed to have a more marked QT prolongation than those without TdP receiving the same I_{Kr} blocking drug and this difference was not related to the dosage of the drug [23]. Patients with drug-induced long QT syndrome are at high risk of recurrent arrhythmias if exposed to the same drug again [24]. The precise reason for the different effects of I_{Kr} blockers is unknown but several factors may be important as discussed below.

Repolarization reserve

One hypothesis to explain the idiosyncratic development of TdP is that normal repolarization is accomplished by multiple, possibly redundant, ion channels, providing a safety reserve for normal repolarization. Thus, in an ordinary situation, the administration of an I_{Kr} blocker does not prolong the QT interval. However, in the presence of an otherwise subclinical impairment in the repolarization mechanisms (i.e., reduced repolarization reserve) [25], for instance in heart failure, which reduces the I_{to} current, the same I_{Kr} blocker may precipitate marked QT prolongation and TdP. The cause of this may be congenital (forme-fruste of congenital LQTS) or acquired (e.g., myocardial infarction, congestive heart failure, etc.). The induction of TdP by a QT-prolonging drug is a patient-specific response [26]. In other words, patients who had a previous history of drug-induced TdP are very likely to develop further episodes of TdP when exposed to any other QT-prolonging drug [27,28].

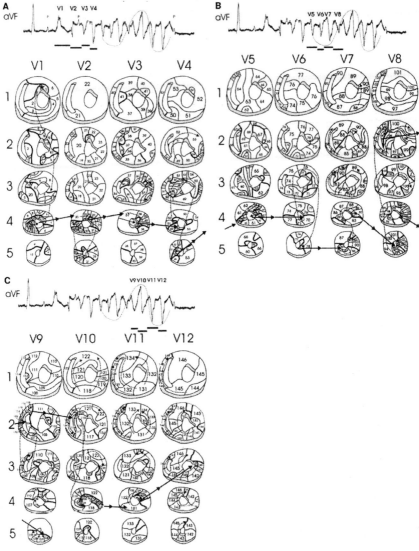

Fig. 2.9 Three-dimensional ventricular activation patterns of the 12-beat nonsustained TdP VT. Functional conduction block is represented in the maps by heavy solid lines. P indicates P waves. The thick bars under the surface ECG lead mark the time intervals covered by each of the tridimensional maps. The V_1 beat arose as a focal subendocardial activity (marked by a star in section 1). All subsequent beats were due to re-entrant excitation. The twisting QRS pattern was more evident in lead aVF during the second half of the VT episode. The transition in QRS axis (between V_7 and V_{10}) correlated with the bifurcation of a predominantly single rotating wave front (scroll) into two separate simultaneous wave fronts rotating around the LV and RV cavities. The final transition in QRS axis (between V_{10} and V_{11}) correlated with the termination of the RV circuit and the reestablishment of a single LV circulating wave front (adapted from [22]).

Forme-fruste of long QT syndrome

In forme-fruste of the long QT syndrome, individuals have mutations in one of the genes known to cause congenital long QT syndrome but little or no QT prolongation at baseline. In these patients, the mutations of the genes render the I_{Kr} or I_{Ks} channels more susceptible to drug blockade, and lower the threshold for the development of QT prolongation and TdP when challenged with an I_{Kr}-blocking drug. Prior to the discovery of genetic mutations responsible for congenital long QT syndrome, Shaw had already reported two patients who might have forme-frustes of the congenital long QT syndrome [29] with recurrent syncope secondary to ventricular fibrillation associated with a normal QT interval, who had been wrongly diagnosed to have epilepsy. One of the patients had normal QT interval at all times whereas the other had normal QT interval with an intermittently abnormal U wave. In both patients, the attacks of ventricular fibrillation were suppressed totally by propranolol. Donger and colleagues described the first missense mutation, $Arg^{555}Cys$, in the C-terminal domain of KVLQT1 gene, which encodes for the α-subunit of a cardiac potassium channel, in families of patients with Romano-Ward congenital long QT syndrome (LQT1-type) [30]. These patients had significantly shorter QTc interval (459 ± 33 ms vs. 480 ± 32 ms, $p = 0.001$), lower risk of syncope (16% vs. 58%, $p < 0.001$) and sudden death (5% vs. 24%, $p < 0.01$) compared with carriers of other mutations at the transmembrane region of the α-subunit. Most of the cardiac events (sudden death or syncope) in these patients were triggered by drugs known to affect repolarization (e.g., disopyramide, mefloquine, diuretics). Thus, the carriers of the C-terminal of KVLQT1 gene have minor or no QT prolongation, are generally devoid of emotion or exercise-induced stress and could not be diagnosed using current diagnostic criteria [31], but may experience drug-induced QT prolongation and arrhythmias.

More recently, Abbott and colleagues identified three missense mutations associated with long QT syndrome in the gene for MiRP1 (MinK-related peptide 1), a small integral membrane β-subunit that assembles with the HERG gene [31]. These mutants form channels open slowly and close rapidly, and thereby diminish potassium currents and cause a clinically silent reduction in potassium current. One variant increased the channel blockade by clarithromycin and was associated with clarithromycin-induced arrhythmia. Thus, it is possible that a genetically inherited reduction in potassium currents can remain clinically silent until it is challenged with additional stressors. Indeed, such patients developed arrhythmic symptoms exclusively after exposure to torsadogenic drugs [30,32].

There have now been some definite reports of clinically silent gene mutations in cardiac ion channels in patients with drug-induced TdP and their relatives [33,34]. Schulze-Bahr and colleagues identified a single nucleotide exchange in the HERG gene (encoding I_{Kr} channel), which resulted in an amino acid alteration within a conserved region of the gene's S2–S3 interdomain, in a female patient with quinidine-induced TdP as well as in her healthy sister who had no QT prolongation but did not receive the medication [33]. Napolitano also reported a female patient with cisapride-induced QT prolongation and TdP, who had a heterogeneous mutation leading to substitution of a highly conserved amino acid in the pore region of KvLQT1 gene (encoding I_{Ks} channel) [34]. Her two otherwise healthy sons with a normal QT interval were also found to be gene carriers. These reports provided further evidence that forme-fruste of long QT syndrome may remain clinically silent until the arrhythmogenic substrate is destabilized, for instance, by an I_{Kr} blocker, and a repetitive arrhythmia may then be easily triggered.

It is also noteworthy that in congenital long QT syndrome with autosomal dominant inheritance, not all carriers of mutant genes have a long QT interval on ECG [35], and not all those affected will have symptoms [36]. Yet, any I_{Kr}-blocking drug may cause life-threatening arrhythmias in these otherwise asymptomatic congenital LQTS patients. Moreover, subtle genetic defects can result in low penetrance of phenotype expression. For instance, Priori and colleagues examined the families with sporadic cases of congenital long QT syndrome (i.e., families in which no members had clinical signs of the conditions apart from the proband) due to missense mutations in the HERG or KVLQT1 genes. They found that among the 46 family members with no clinical long QT syndrome, 33% were identified to be gene carriers [37]. The penetrance rate was 25% and conventional diagnostic criteria only had a sensitivity of 38% in identifying the carriers of these genetic defects. Recently, an autosomal recessive inheritance of long QT syndrome without deafness has been described [38]. Thus, these silent gene carriers with genetic mutation for congenital long QT syndrome may have no or different phenotypical manifestation but are at risk of developing TdP if exposed to QT-prolonging drugs, as well as passing the genetic defects to their offspring. These findings have enormous implications, especially in drug-induced proarrhythmia, since they suggest that silent gene carriers with mild mutations are probably not as rare as is commonly assumed although at present, forme-fruste of congenital long QT syndrome only accounts for a minority of patients with drug-induced TdP. Despite the fact that many genetic defects are yet to be identified, large-scale screening of patients before prescribing QT-prolonging drugs may become possible and necessary. Whether these patients are at risk of developing other acquired forms of QT prolongation, for instance, during myocardial ischaemia, remains to be seen.

Other risk factors
Apart from the congenital long QT syndrome and drugs, other risk factors that can affect repolarization include:
• Organic heart disease (e.g., ischaemic heart disease, congestive heart failure, dilated cardiomyopathy, hypertrophic cardiomyopathy, myocarditis and Kawasaki syndrome).
• Sinus bradycardia, atrioventricular and sinoatrial blocks.

- Drug-related factors (e.g., narrow therapeutic window, a multiplicity of pharmacological actions and inhibition and induction of cytochrome P450 enzymes, polypharmacy).
- Electrolyte abnormalities (e.g., hypokalaemia (by far the commonest), hypocalcaemia, hypomagnesaemia).
- Female gender.
- Diabetes mellitus.
- Anorexia nervosa.
- Hepatic impairment/cirrhosis.
- Intracranial hemorrhage.
- Hypothyroidism.
- Liquid protein diet.

References

1 Tan HL, Hou CJY, Lauer MR, Sung RJ. Electrophysiologic mechanism of the long QT interval syndrome and torsades de pointes. *Ann Intern Med* 1995; 122: 701–14.
2 Priori SG, Barhanin J, Hauer RN *et al*. Genetic and molecular basis of cardiac arrhythmias: impact on clinical management part III. *Circulation* 1999; 99 (5): 674–81.
3 Sicouri S, Antzelevitch C. A subpopulation of cells with unique electrophysiological properties in the deep subepicardium of canine ventricle. The M cell. *Cir Res* 1991; 68: 1729–41.
4 Antzelevitch C, Davidenko JM, Sicouri S *et al*. Quinidine-induced early afterdepolarization and triggered activity. *J Electrophysiol* 1989; 3: 323–38.
5 Carmeliet E. Voltage- and time-dependent block of the delayed K current in cardiac myocytes by dofetilide. *J Pharmacol Exp Ther* 1992; 262: 809–17.
6 Liu DW, Antzelevitch C. Characteristics of the delayed rectifier current (I_{Kr} and I_{Ks}) in canine ventricular epicardial, midmyocardial, and endocardial myocytes. A weaker I_{Ks} contributes to the longer action potential of the M cell. *Circ Res* 1995; 76: 351–65.
7 Antzelevitch C, Sicouri S. Clinical relevance of cardiac arrhythmias generated by afterdepolarization: role of M cells in the generation of U wave, triggered activity, and torsades de pointes. *J Am Coll Cardiol* 1994; 23: 259–77.
8 Liu DW, Antzelevitch C. Characteristics of the delayed rectifier current (I_{Kr} and I_{Ks}) in canine ventricular epicardial, midmyocardial, and endocardial myocytes. A weaker I_{Ks} contributes to the longer action potential of the M cell. *Cir Res* 1995; 76: 351–65.
9 Shimizu W, Antzelevitch C. Cellular and ionic basis for T-wave alternans under long QT conditions. *Circulation* 1999; 10: 244–60.
10 Camm AJ, Janse MJ, Roden DM, Rosen MR, Cinca J, Cobbe SM. Congenital and acquired long QT syndrome. *Eur Heart J* 2000; 21: 1232–7.
11 Kay GN, Plumb VJ, Arciniegas JG *et al*. Torsades de pointes: The long-short initiating sequence and other clinical features: Observations in 32 patients. *J Am Coll Cardiol* 1983; 2: 806–17.
12 Haverkamp W, Shenasa M, Borggrefe M, Breithardt G 1995 In: Zipes, DP, Jalife, J, eds. *Cardiac Electrophysiology: from Cell to Bedside*, 2nd edn. Philadelphia: W.B. Saunders, pp. 885–9.

13 Roden DM, Woosley RL, Primm RK. Incidence and clinical features of the quinidine–associated long QT syndrome: Implications for patient care. *Am Heart J* 1986; 111: 1088–93.

14 Roden DM, Thompson KA, Hoffman BF, Woosley RL. Clinical features and basic mechanisms of quinidine-induced arrhythmias. *J Am Coll Cardiol* 1986; 8: 73A–78A.

15 Jackman WM, Friday KJ, Anderson JL, Aliot EM, Clark M, Lazzara R. The long QT syndromes. a critical review, new clinical observations and a unifying hypothesis. *Prog Cardiovasc Dis* 1988; 31: 115–72.

16 Brugada P, Wellens HJJ. Early afterdepolarization. role in conduction block, "prolonged repolarization-dependent reexcitation", and tachyarrhythmias in the human heart. *Pacing Clin Electrophysiol* 1985; 8: 889–96.

17 El-Sherif N, Caref EB, Chinushi M, Restivo M. Mechanism of arrhythmogenicity of the short-long sequence that precedes ventricular tachyarrhythmias in the long QT syndrome. *J Am Coll Cardiol* 1999; 33: 1415–23.

18 Wiener I, Kunkes S, Rubib D, Kupersmith J, Packer M, Pitchon R, Schweitzer P. Effects of sudden change in cycle length on human atrial, atrioventricular nodal and ventricular refractory periods. *Circulation* 1981; 64: 245–8.

19 Nattel S, Quantz MA. Pharmacological response of quinidine induced early afterdepolarization in canine cardiac Purkinje fibres: insights into underlying ionic mechanisms. *Cardiovasc Res* 1988; 22: 808–17.

20 Fabiota A, Coumel P. Torsades de pointes, a quarter of a century later: a tribute to Dr. F. Dessertenne. *Cardiovasc Drug Ther* 1991; 5: 167–70.

21 Malik M, Camm AJ. Possible pathophysiology of torsade de pointes evaluated by a realistic heart computer model. *Cardiovas Res* 1986; 20:436–43.

22 El-Sherif N, Chinushi M, Caref EB, Restivo M. Electrophysiological mechanism of the characteristic electrocardiographic morphology of torsade de pointes tachyarrhythmias in the long–QT syndrome: detailed analysis of ventricular tridimensional activation patterns. *Circulation* 1997; 96 (12): 4392–9.

23 Houltz B, Darpo B, Edvardsson N et al. Electrocardiographic and clinical predictors of torsades de pointes induced by almokalant infusion in patients with chronic atrial fibrillation or flutter: a prospective study. *Pacing Clin Electrophysiol* 1998; 21 (5): 1044–57.

24 Jackman WM, Friday KJ, Anderson JL, Aliot EM, Clark M, Lazzara R. The long QT syndrome. a critical review, new clinical observations and a unifying hypothesis. *Prog Cardiovasc Dis* 1988; 31: 115–72.

25 Roden D. Taking the idio out of idiosyncratic – predicting torsades de pointes. *Pacing Clin Electrophysiol* 1998; 21: 1029–34.

26 Haverkamp W, Breithardt G, Camm AJ et al. The potential for QT prolongation and proarrhythmia by nonantiarrhythmic drugs: clinical and regulatory implications. *Eur Heart J* 2000; 21: 1216–31.

27 Soffer J, Dreifus LS, Michelson EL. Polymorphous ventricular tachycardia associated with normal and long QT interval. *Am J Cardiol* 1982; 49: 2021–9.

28 Wald RW, Waxman MB, Colman JM. Torsades de pointes ventricular tachycardia. A complication of disopyramide shared with quinidine. *J Electrocardiol* 1981; 14: 301–7.

29 Shaw TR. Recurrent ventricular fibrillation associated with normal QT intervals. *Q J Med* 1981; 50 (200): 451–62.

30 Donger C, Denjoy I, Berthet M et al. KVLQT1 C-terminal missense mutation causes a forme fruste long QT syndrome. *Circulation* 1997; 96: 2778–81.

31 Schwartz PJ, Moss AJ, Vincent GM, Crampton RS. Diagnostic criteria for the long QT syndrome: an update. *Circulation* 1993; 88: 782–4.

32 Abbott GW, Sesti F, Splawski I, Buck ME, Lehmann MH, Timothy KW, Keating MT, Goldstein SA. MiRP1 forms IKr potassium channels with HERG and is associated with cardiac arrhythmia. *Cell* 1999; 97 (2): 175–87.

33 Schulze-Bahr E, Haverkamp W, Hördt M, Wedekind H, Borggrefe M. Do mutations in cardiac ion channel genes predispose to drug-induced (acquired) long QT syndrome? *Circulation* 1997; 96 (Suppl. I): (Abstract): I-211.

34 Napolitano C, Schwartz P, Brown AM *et al.* Evidence for a cardiac ion channel mutation underlying drug-induced QT prolongation and life-threatening arrhythmias. *J Cardiovasc Electrophysiol* 2000; 11 (6): 691–6.

35 Vincent GM, Timothy KW, Leppert M, Keating M. The spectrum of symptoms and QT intervals in carriers of the gene fro the long QT syndrome. *N Engl J Med* 1992; 327: 846–52.

36 Zareba W, Moss AJ, Schwartz PJ. Influence of the genotype on the clinical course of the long QT syndrome. *N Engl J Med* 1998; 339: 960–5.

37 Priori SG, Napolitano C, Schwartz PJ. Low penetrance in the long QT syndrome. Clinical impact. *Circulation* 1999; 99: 529–33.

38 Priori SG, Schwartz PJ, Napolitano Bianchi L, Dennis A, De Fusco M, Brown AM, Casari G. A recessive variant of the Romano–Ward long QT syndrome? *Circulation* 1998; 97: 2420–5.

CHAPTER 3

Measurement of QT interval and repolarization assessment

Measurement of QT interval

The QT interval conceptually represents the duration from the onset of depolarization to the completion of repolarization. On a standard ECG, it is measured from the beginning of the QRS complex (or RS complex if there is no Q wave) to the end of the T wave. The onset of the QRS complex is usually easily defined (although frequent exceptions exist) and the most difficult aspect of the methodology of measuring the QT interval is the identification of the T wave offset, which in turn is influenced by the T wave amplitude, presence of a U wave and baseline noise. Several techniques have been used previously but all approaches are associated with potential inaccuracies. The most frequently cited method is that proposed by Surawicz and Knoebel [1]. In this method, the ECG is recorded at a paper speed of 50 mm/s and at gain of 20 mm/mV using a multichannel recorder capable of simultaneous recording of all 12 leads. A tangent line to the steepest part of the descending portion of the T wave is drawn and the intercept between the tangent line and the isoelectric line is defined as the end of T wave [2]. While this method is cited by almost every laboratory involved in QT interval measurement, it is not necessarily always precisely followed. Precision of drawing the tangent is highly dubious when performed by hand and at best problematic if supported by a computer. Tiny noise perturbations in the ECG signal can easily influence the localization of the "steepest part" of the descending point of the T wave and different interpolation techniques used to define the tangent may lead to surprisingly different results. The seminal article on this "tangent" method by Lepschkin and Surawicz seems also more frequently quoted than carefully read. The method of drawing the tangent to the descending part of the T wave was proposed as one of the possibilities to be used in cases when much simpler determination of the return to baseline fails because the very end of the T wave is blurred by U wave, noise, electrocardiographic baseline wonder, etc. It can be easily seen that this method depends not only on the shape of the descending part of the T wave but is also highly influenced by impressions in the determination of the baseline.

As with every electrocardiographic measurement, the duration of QT interval assessed in one single cardiac beat is not necessarily very relevant. Although the changes in RR interval due to respiratory arrhythmia do not have any meaningful effect on the QT interval duration (as discussed in more detail later) there are respiration driven changes in the morphology of the T wave. Therefore, several measurements taken from different cardiac cycles of the same short-term electrocardiogram need to be averaged to obtain a representative duration of the QT interval at any given time. The influence of such averaging on the precision of the reading of the interval naturally depends on the quality of the electrocardiogram as well as on the precision of the measurement technology itself. The more beats are averaged, the greater the precision and a broad consensus exists that no fewer than 3 beats should be measured. Increased precision frequently requires greater number of interval readings to be averaged, such as 5 or even more. In standard 10-second short-term electrocardiograms recorded at stable conditions, there is no appreciable change in the QT interval duration during the recording. While it is frequently believed that the cardiac cycles used for averaging of QT interval measurements should be consecutive, this assumption is unfounded. In a short-term electrocardiogram, it is frequently not only more precise but also easier to select the least noise polluted cardiac cycles for the measurement.

There are numerous sources of potential inaccuracy in QT interval measurement ranging from the identification of the T wave and the distinction of physiological and pathological U wave to the technical details of measurement technology and selection of electrocardiographic leads.

Moreover, since the duration of QT interval depends on many physiological factors, among which the heart rate is most dominant, it is usually the heart rate corrected QT interval that is used in the assessment of QT interval changes such as those related to drug treatment. The impression of heart rate correction is surprisingly frequently much greater than the impression of the measurement of the source interval itself. In studies in which substantial precision is needed, mainly when assessing drug effects on the duration of the QT interval, particular attention needs to be given to heart rate correction. It is senseless to try to improve the measurement of the original QT interval only to spoil it later by gross errors in heart rate correction.

The identification of T wave offset and the presence of U waves

A particular problem of QT interval measurement is the definition of the end of the T wave despite a perfectly formed T wave and the distinction between T and U waves. The shape of the T wave itself can be very variable [3] [Fig. 3.1], and problems can arise when the T wave is flat, bifid, biphasic, or when the T and U waves cannot be distinguished. Furthermore, during the offset of the T wave, the slow-moving deflection of the T wave can be contaminated with noise. Hence, not all ECG leads have measurable QT intervals. Occasionally, electrocardiograms are found in which none or only very few leads are measurable despite a reasonable quality of the recording. Cases of that kind are always problematic and we shall discuss them in more detail in the section on the selection of leads of measurement.

The origin of T and U waves remains disputed. Theories that attributed the U wave to the repolarization of the Purkinje fibers [4] or to a mechano-electrical

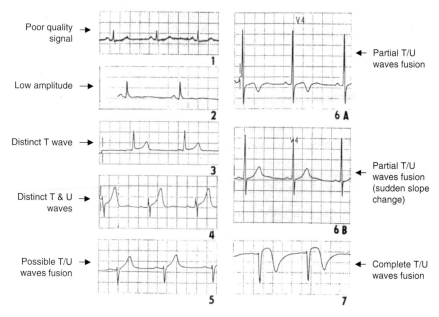

Fig. 3.1 Multiple complex morphology of T wave (adapted from [3]).

mechanism [5] were superseded by the M-cell theory of Antzelevich *et al.* as discussed in Chapter 2. However, later experiments by the same group showed that a "pathologically augmented U wave" or "T–U complex" may in fact be a result of a prolonged bi-phasic T wave with an interrupted ascending or descending limb [6]. Measurement is even less reliable for certain T–U patterns, e.g., when the T wave is flat or inverted and the U wave augmented. Many conditions can produce U waves especially congenital and drug–induced long QT syndromes, which can obscure the T wave offset. The measurement is made difficult if a U wave is present which merges with the T wave (commonly seen in congenital long QT syndrome) to produce a bizarrely shaped T wave such that the end of the T wave (or T–U wave) may have a higher amplitude than the beginning of the wave. A substantial variability of the measurement often results from complex morphology repolarization patterns being classified differently by different observers [3].

The electrophysiologic mechanisms that are responsible for the common "physiological" U waves are probably different from those leading to abnormal U waves, e.g., those seen in acquired long QT syndrome (Fig. 3.2a,b). It seems reasonable to propose that all electrocardiographic signals originating from repolarization of the ventricular myocardium should belong to the T wave. In this respect, the concept of bi-phasic and other unusually shaped T waves is more appropriate than a distinction between the T wave and an augmented U wave that may lead to serious underestimation of

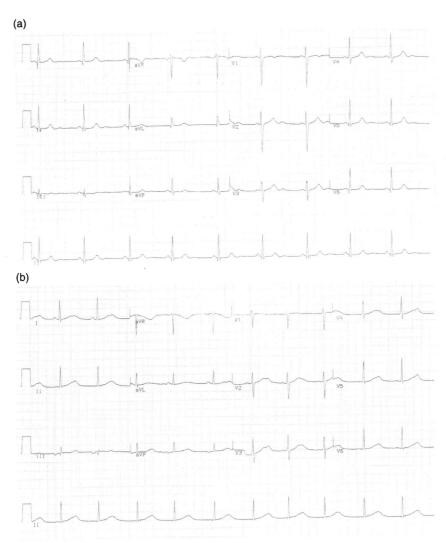

Fig. 3.2 (a) ECG of a healthy subject with physiological U wave, best seen on the anterior chest leads. (b) Pathological U wave on the ECG of a patient with congenital long QT syndrome.

the QT interval. Augmented pathological U waves may be the only sign of adverse repolarization changes, e.g., in the ECG recordings of patients taking mibefradil [7]. However, a pattern resembling an augmented U wave may also originate from slow after-depolarizations. Distinction of such patterns from bizarre T waves may be very difficult. On the other hand, they also indicate the same proarrhythmic danger as do bizarre T wave shapes and/or a prolonged QT interval. It is also important to note that QT interval is a function of T wave duration. Therefore, the presence of a merged T/U wave complex signifies abnormal ventricular repolarization, and the exclusion of a U wave from a T/U complex for QT interval measurement will decrease the power of the QT interval measurement to reflect any abnormality of repolarization and may be misleading. Therefore, it is usual to include an abnormal U wave in the QT interval measurement if it is part of the T/U complex. In all cases that are difficult to reconcile, augmented U waves should be preferably included into the T wave. The U wave should probably not be incorporated in the QT measurement when there is a clear distinction between the T wave and an obviously "physiological" U wave of small amplitude. Such U waves have no pathological significance and can be safely ignored.

In 1952, Lepeschkin and Surawicz [2] described and classified various patterns of T and U wave merging and suggested methods for determining the end of the T wave when "buried" within the U wave (Fig. 3.3). They showed that, depending on the pattern of T–U wave amalgamation, either the intersection of the tangent to the steepest downslope of the T wave with the isoelectric line, or the nadir between the T and the U waves is closest to the "real" T wave end.

Some investigators tried to improve the method of defining the T wave offset/end by increasing the amplifier gain and/or reducing the paper

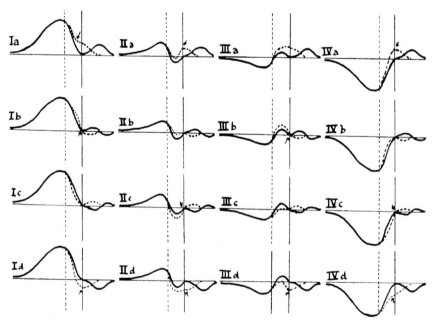

Fig. 3.3 Classification of various patterns of merged T and U wave and suggested methods for determining the end of the T wave when "buried" within the U wave (Adapted from Lepeschkin and Surawicz [2]).

speed. However, these are potentially flawed. Murray *et al.* demonstrated that QT interval measurements were significantly longer by 8 ms for a doubling of the gain, and by 11 ms and 16 ms when the paper speed was reduced from 100 to 50 mm/s and 50–25 mm/s, respectively [8]. Thus, any comparison between QT intervals must ensure that similar amplifier gain and paper speed are used between studies.

Optimal lead used

Traditionally, lead II has been used frequently for QT interval measurement because in this lead, the vectors of repolarization usually result in a long single wave rather than discrete T and U waves. It has also been reported that in healthy electrocardiograms (but not those with repolarization abnormalities) lead II most frequently contains the longest QT interval. More recent experience with digital electrocardiograms precisely measured in every measurable lead suggests that the selection of lead II for measurement is highly problematic. Not only does the maximum QT interval very frequently occur in different leads but also is the distribution of the leads containing the maximum QT interval duration different study to study (Fig. 3.4). The measurement of QT interval in lead II is therefore based more on a poor tradition than on any solid reasoning. Allowing an alternate lead, such

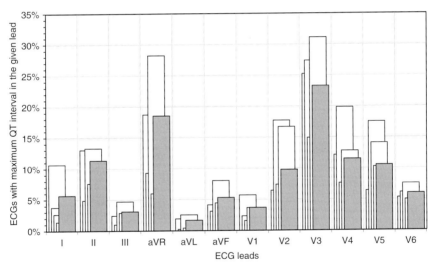

Fig. 3.4 Distribution of the maximum QT interval among 12-leads in electrocardiograms recorded in 4 clinical studies, each containing in excess of 2000 digital electrocardiograms measured in each lead using an accurate technology that included blinded measurement by multiple observers with subsequent reconciliation. The front grey bars show the average incidence of the maximum QT interval in any given lead, the overlaid open bars show the distribution in the four separate studies. Lead II contained the maximum QT interval in less than 15% of recordings of each study. Moreover, the distribution of the maximum QT durations varied highly from study to study and thus, extrapolations of this kind from one series of electrocardiograms are not necessarily valid in a different series of recordings. (Malik M., 2003, unpublished data.)

as V_2, when lead II is unreadable, is even more inadequate because for instance, a drug that affects the T wave may render one or other lead unreadable, allowing only an inappropriate comparison of different leads, before and after drug administration.

Many clinical studies used various other criteria including maximum QT interval in any limb lead [9], maximum QT interval in any of the 12 leads [10], lead with most distinct (tallest) T wave [11] or lead AVL where U wave is usually isoelectric [12]. Others proposed that the mean values for the QT interval measured using multiple leads recorded simultaneously might be more appropriate. Clearly, different lead selection criteria would result in very different estimates of QT interval [13]. Occasionally, electrocardiograms are found in which either none or very few leads have the QT interval measurable (Fig. 3.5). Tracings of that kind are best excluded from any precise study since the possibility cannot be excluded that the measurable lead contains an isoelectric terminal portion of the T wave that leads to an artificially shortened QT interval measurement. Approximate measurements based on guesswork (including, for instance, cases when electrocardiographic laboratories claim that they can measure small amplitude T waves that on paper printed electrocardiograms are only visible when using a magnifying glass) should always be avoided because they always introduce gross inaccuracies. (In standard paper printed electrocardiograms, the width of the line of the tracing is approximately 10 ms even if the tracing is of good technical quality.) It is also advocated that the so-called quasi-orthogonal system, i.e., the measurement of the QT interval from the earliest Q wave onset in quasi-orthogonal leads I, aVF, and V2, to the latest T wave offset in these three leads, might provide a more comprehensive assessment of the

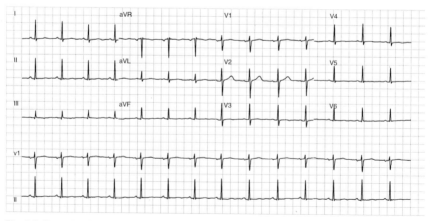

Fig. 3.5 Example of an electrocardiogram in which reasonable precision of QT interval measurement can only be achieved in lead V2. While very small deflections of the T wave are visible in some other leads (including lead II) their measurement is not possible with any meaningful precision.

QT interval irrespective of the morphology of the vectorcardiographic loop of the T wave. Others argue that the quasi-orthogonal system is not necessarily truly orthogonal under all circumstances and that changes in the cardiac axis and in ventricular gradient may distort the results of the quasi-orthogonal measurement. Moreover, this method requires that all the three quasi-orthogonal leads are measurable. Experience shows that this is frequently not the case because lead aVF belongs to those in which the T wave is often isoelectric (in around 20% of recordings).

When digital ECG recordings are obtained, truly orthogonal XYZ leads may be reconstructed if not directly recorded. The measurement in the orthogonal XYZ system (again, from the earliest onset to the latest offset) would overcome some of the problems of the quasi-orthogonal system but the present experience is too limited to allow solid recommendations.

It has been well recognized that the QT interval can vary considerably between leads within the same ECG. Such variation is due to the timing of the end of the T wave, rather than the onset of the QRS complex and is considerably greater than the variability due to cycles, observers or measurement error [13]. One explanation for this inter-lead variation is that it represents differing orientation of different leads to the repolarization vector. A lead at 90° to the vector would therefore become isoelectric before a lead in the line of the vector. A hypothesis that the inter-lead variation is due to spatial (regional) differences in repolarization, a phenomenon described as QT dispersion (see below), has now been abandoned [14]. Cowan and colleagues examined the optimal lead for QT interval measurement [13]. They argued that if inter-lead QT variation is due to differing orientations to a single repolarization vector, then, the best representation of the duration of electrical systole must be the maximum QT interval in any lead. Since the maximum QT interval can occur in any lead, it is therefore necessary to measure all 12 leads if this definition is adopted. However, this is not realistic in routine clinical practice as well as in large (e.g., Phase III and Phase IV) clinical trials. An approximation to maximum QT interval should be adopted. They had shown in their study that leads V2 or V3 provided the closest approximation to maximum QT interval and recommend that one of these leads should be chosen as the standard lead for QT measurement.

Still, while based on reasonable theoretical considerations, the precision with which the maximum QT interval can be measured is questionable. As with any other measurement, assessing extremes magnifies measurement imprecision and leads to data of questionable properties. Average or, preferably, median QT interval duration of different measured leads has, for simple mathematical reasons, much superior stability.

Therefore, some authorities advocate the use of median duration of QT interval. In such a case, the QT interval in all 12 leads of the ECGs are measured and the median duration of the QT intervals of all the measurable leads is taken in the assumption that the drug effect on ventricular repolarization is similar in all myocardial regions, especially in healthy subjects.

Practical experience (Malik M., unpublished data) also shows that conclusions of drug-related QT interval changes based on median QT interval do not differ from those based on maximum QT interval that has been measured under a strict quality control. Once the electrocardiograms are obtained digitally, it is also not necessary to measure each lead separately. Providing the isoelectric line is properly defined in each lead, images of different leads can be superimposed on the same isoelectric line and displayed together. Experience shows that in such a display, the identification of both QRS onset and T wave offset is easier than in separate leads. Problems resulting from the isoelectric projection of terminal part of T wave in some leads are avoided since the difference between different leads is easily visible. Likewise, distinction between the T wave and physiological U wave is made more obvious. At the same time, since the definition of isoelectric baseline and removal of baseline wander can be computerized in most cases, this type of display of electrocardiogram can be made practically without any manual involvement. Hence, measuring the images of superimposed ECG leads is not more difficult than measuring one single lead while the precision of the assessment of the true duration of the QT interval is greatly improved (Fig. 3.6).

Manual vs. automated method

The ideal method used to measure the QT interval has been a subject of debate. While most modern electrocardiographs report an automatic

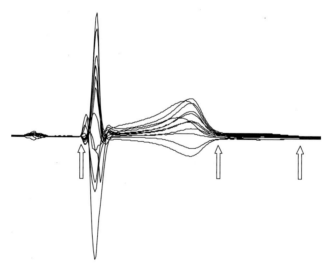

Fig. 3.6 Images of 12-lead recording of one cardiac cycle superimposed on the same isoelectric axis. It is easy to detect not only the onset QRS complex and the offset of T wave but also the offset of the very low amplitude physiological U wave (all marked by arrows). It is also easy to see that in some leads, the terminal part of the T wave projects into the isoelectric line while in all other leads, the T wave terminates literally at the same time. Manual measurement of this pattern are not more complicated (actually frequently easier) than similar measurements of any separate lead.

measurement of the QT interval, these automatically obtained values are usually correct only in normal noise-free electrocardiograms in which the pattern of the T wave is well defined. Morphologic abnormalities of the T wave, noise in the signal as well as confusion between the T and U wave may easily invalidate automatic measurements (Fig. 3.7). While it is possibly not surprising that gross noise pollution (such as that seen in lead V1 in Fig. 3.7b) or confusion between T wave and U wave (e.g., Fig. 3.7a) may lead to substantial imprecision in fully automatic reading of the QT interval, the assessment by electrocardiograph is frequently sensitive even to noise pollution by the standard alternating current which should be expected and dealt with appropriately in equipment of any reasonable quality (Fig. 3.8). Occasionally, bizarre automatic QT interval readings are reported by electrocardiographs even for tracings that are perfectly normal and noise free (Fig. 3.9). For all these reasons, it has been suggested that automated methods yield less

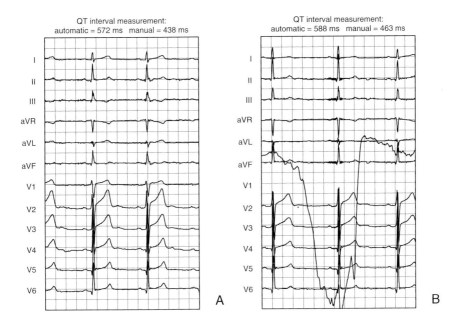

Fig. 3.7 Two examples of errors in computer measurement of the QT interval in 12 lead electrocardiograms. The automatic reading of both electrocardiograms were obtained by the ECG Research Workstation by Marquette GE, which is one of the leading technical systems for electrocardiogram processing. In the electrocardiogram in panel A shows, the computer program was probably confused by the physiologic U waves (note lead V_2). The manual reading of the QT interval was 438 ms while the automatic reading showed 572 ms. In panel B, the noise in the limb leads and loss of signal in V_1 probably contributed to the erroneous automatic reading of 588 ms while the manual reading was 463 ms. Each square of the display corresponds to 200 ms/500 μV.

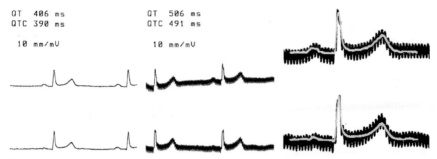

Fig. 3.8 Errors in automatic measurements by electrocardiograph due to (presumably) pollution by alternating current. The left and middle panel show electrocardiographic images which differed in their automatic measurement of QT interval by 100 ms. The right panel shows a superimposition of the QRS and T wave images of the left and middle panel. It is obvious that the duration of the uncorrected QT interval was practically the same in both cases.

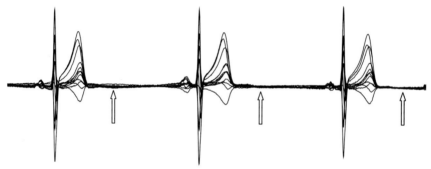

Fig. 3.9 Superimposition of all 12-leads of a perfectly normal and almost noise free electrocardiogram. The manual reading the QT interval was 404 ms while the automatic measurement showed 674 ms. Assuming that the detection of the QRS onset was correct in the automatic measurement, the arrows show where the T wave offset was measured. The reasons for such a substantial failure of a modern electrocardiograph handling digital data is not obvious.

accurate results than manual methods [15], and no simple automatic algorithm has so far been shown to be sufficiently precise and robust to satisfy the accuracy required in the assessment of cardiac safety of a drug. Some workers, however, reported that both automatic and manual methods (using digitizing board) provided similar values [16]. With the manual method, the recording technology plays an important role for the precision of QT interval measurement. In the past, electrocardiograms were normally recorded only on paper using most frequently the standard 25 mm/s paper speed and 10 mm/mV gain. From ECGs recorded in this way, the QT interval was sometime measured using procedures of questionable precision including the use of hand-held callipers. More recently, paper-printed electrocardiograms have been measured on a digitizing board, in the belief that the technical precision of the digitizing equipment can be matched by human operators. Unfortunately such beliefs are not justified and measurement of paper-printed electrocardiograms using digitizing boards may lead to very substantial errors [17]. Errors of up to 3 mm (that is $\pm$ 120 ms at 25 mm/s) in repeated measurements were reported [17]. With the manual method using a digitizing board, Kautzner and colleagues examined the short- and long-term reproducibility of QT interval measurement in healthy subjects using a digitizing board with a 0.1-mm resolution [3]. Using this method, the measurement of the QT interval from standard ECG recordings was feasible and not operator dependent, with an interobserver relative error of <4%. The duration of the QT interval was stable and its short-term (1 day) and long-term (1 week and 1 month) reproducibility was high with an intrasubject relative error of <6%. However, accurate manual QT interval measurement using a digitizing board requires considerable experience in using the tool, as well as identifying the T wave offset. Such an error is particularly true when measuring QT intervals in myocardial infarction patients where large errors have been reported between observers not specifically experienced in QT interval measurement [18].

Not infrequently clinical research organizations involved in the QT interval measurement from electrocardiograms in drug studies employ operators without proper, if any, training (Fig. 3.10). Some regulators therefore argue that all QT interval measurements related to drug safety assessment should be performed only by cardiologists. This is not because cardiologists would be expected to be more accurate and/or more systematic than trained cardiac technicians, but because the electrophysiologic understanding of ECG signals should guarantee proper handling of unusual and/or complicated cases in which gross error and omissions otherwise usually appear.

The selection of the beats to be measured needs also to be performed carefully. For instance, beats following the compensatory pause of an atrial or ventricular premature beat should be avoided because the T wave is known to be frequently abnormal in these beats [19].

Several measurement algorithms have been proposed to determine the end of the T wave automatically. It is noteworthy that when using automated method manufacturers use different algorithms to calculate intervals and this must be considered when comparing results from different computerized systems. Mclaughlin and colleagues examined the reproducibility of four different algorithms, namely: threshold method (TH); differential threshold method (DTH); slope method (SL) and; peak slope method (PSI) (Fig. 3.11), in measuring the QT interval [20,21]. For TH method, the T wave offset was determined as the interception of a threshold level with the T wave. In DTH method, the T wave offset was defined as the interception of a threshold level and the differential of the T wave. For both TH and DTH methods, the threshold levels were calculated as a fraction, in the range of 5–15%, of the amplitude of the T wave or differential T wave, respectively. The final two algorithms were based on slope features. In SL method, then

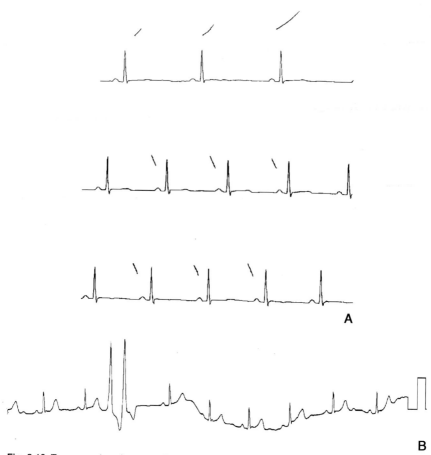

Fig. 3.10 Two examples of poor quality of manual QT interval measurement are shown. The tracings in panel A are of lead II from serial electrocardiograms of the same subject recorded during a Phase I study. In each of these leads, the QT intervals in three cardiac complexes should have been measured. The ticks were made by an operator identifying complexes that he/she measured. Note that these include cardiac cycles in which no T wave could have been identified. In the tracing from a different Phase I study shown in panel B, the QT interval was measured correctly but the operator included the couplet of extrasystoles into the calculation of heart rate (dividing the interval between the first and last sinus rhythm QRS complex by 9 RR intervals). This led to overestimation of heart rate and to an artificially prolonged QTc interval. In both cases, the reported QT and RR values were recorded in the study database and subsequently constituted substantial outliers with a considerable QTc interval prolongation.

end of T wave was taken as the interception of an isoelectric level and a line tangential to the point of maximum T wave slope. The PSI method calculated the end of T wave as the interception point between an isoelectric level and the line that passes through the peak of the T wave and the point of maximum T wave slope. They found that the mean QT interval measurement,

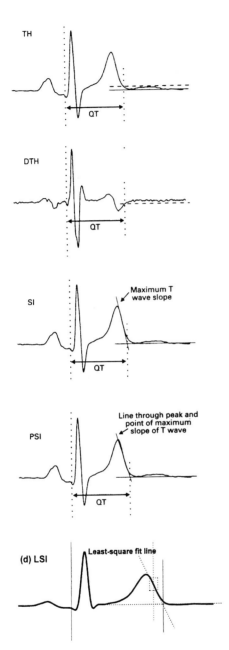

a) The threshold method (TH): the interception of a threshold level and the T wave.

b) The differential threshold method (DTH): the interception of a threshold level and the differential of the T wave.

c) The slope method (SL): the interception of a line tangential to the point of maximum T wave slope and isoelectric level

d) The peak slope method (PSI): interception of an isoelectric level and the line passing through the peak and point of maximum slope of the T wave.

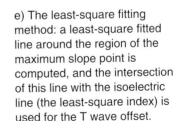

e) The least-square fitting method: a least-square fitted line around the region of the maximum slope point is computed, and the intersection of this line with the isoelectric line (the least-square index) is used for the T wave offset.

Fig. 3.11 The main algorithms used for determining the end of the T wave include (modified from [20–21], with permission from the BMJ Publishing Group; and [22]).

particularly with TH and DTH methods, was extremely variable depending on the filtering bandwidths, isoelectric and threshold levels, and recommended that TH method should not be used for clinical purposes for the reason mentioned. Furthermore, slope-based algorithms had better reproducibility than threshold-based methods due to more stable point of intersection with the isoelectric line. However, the slope method may theoretically cut off the terminal portion of the T wave and reduce its accuracy for QT interval measurement. Xue *et al.* also showed that slope-based methods in general had better reproducibility than the threshold methods in determining T wave offset although they used a least-square fitting slope-based algorithm in determining the T wave offset [22]. In the least-square fitting method, a least-square fitted line around the region of the maximum slope point is computed, and the intersection of this line with the isoelectric line (the least-square index) is used for the T wave offset.

Most recently, it has been realised that the majority of the problems with automatic measurement are mainly caused by the failure of simple automatic algorithms (such as those discussed previously) in electrocardiograms with T wave morphologies that contradict the assumption of the elementary methods. (Practically for every elementary method, an electrocardiogram can be found in which the morphology of the T wave and/or of the T/U patterns makes the results of the simple computer algorithm bizarrely wrong.) Progress has been made in combining a large of number of elementary methods and establishing the relationship between their results and measurements made with a careful manual technology. From such comparisons, proper combinations of elementary methods can be derived and used prospectively. It seems that in this way, both reliable and fully automatic measurements will be made possible in the very near future.

QT interval can also be measured from Holter ECG recording. There seem to be several advantages that this technique provides. Most frequently, the advantage is considered on measuring the QT interval over a wide range of heart rates, thus allowing direct comparison of the QT intervals at various heart rates without heart rate correction. However, as discussed further, there is a considerable time hysteresis between a change in heart rate and the subsequent change in QT interval [23]. Thus beat-to-beat analysis of QT/RR pairs that uses the immediate preceding RR interval cannot reliably reflect the heart rate influence on ventricular repolarization. The use of Holter recording to assess the QT dynamicity analysis will possibly adjust for such a shortfall. There is also a serious principal limitation of the so-called "bin method" that compares QT intervals that occur at the same heart rate before and after intervention. When used with drugs that change heart rate, the same heart rates before and during treatment occur at different stages of autonomic modulations that have an appreciable effect on the QT interval duration on their own. For instance when investigating a drug and accelerates heart rate independently of the autonomic system, the same heart rates on and off treatment occur in episodes that on treatment have greater vagal influence while off treatment greater sympathetic influence on the QT interval. Since sympathetic overdrive shortens the duration of QT interval, the off treatment recordings will have shorter QT interval durations at the same heart rate not because of drug induced QT interval prolongation but because of the disparity in the autonomic background on and off treatment. False-positive (and similarly false-negative) findings may be obtained in this way.

Moreover, there are other technical limitations linked to the use of long-term Holter recordings. For instance, there are a large number of complexes needed to be analyzed, a reduced number of leads available for analysis and the frequent presence of noise in the recording [24]. Newer digital Holter recorders that are capable of recording 12-lead ECGs over 24 h are now available commercially and will overcome the problem of limited number of leads with three-channels recordings. Furthermore, the normal ranges of QT interval using this technique may differ from those established for standard 12-lead recordings [25]. Depending on the leads selected, Holter measurements of QT intervals could range from 55 ms longer to 100 ms shorter (lead V1), or from 62 ms longer to 42 ms shorter (lead V5) than values obtained using standard 12-lead ECG [25].

With advances in electrocardiographic equipment, the possibility of recording 12-lead electrocardiograms digitally has occurred. Digital recordings may be displayed on computer screens with a substantial magnification (up to 10 times the paper display) and measured with computer driven on-screen callipers, the precision of which corresponds to the sampling frequency of the electrocardiograms (usually 500 Hz, i.e., one sample every 2 ms leading to a theoretic measurement precision of $\pm$ 1 ms). Even more importantly, the on-screen measurement allows the whole history of the measurement to be stored, that is not only the duration of QT interval is reported but also the precise positions of the Q-onset and T-offset are localized within the electrocardiograms. Because of these advantages, on-screen measurement is also frequently considered with scanned paper-recorded electrocardiograms. Systems also exist for conversion of scanned paper-recorded signals into digital electrocardiograms. However, scanning paper records should be restricted only to evaluation of previously recorded data that do not exist in another form.

At present, the quality of automatic QT measurement for the assessment of drug-induced QT prolongation is frequently poor and substantial measurement errors occur. The solution is not even in the combination of simple automatic and manual measurement, particularly when manual measurement is restricted to the outliers in the database of automatically generated data. In such a case, one may reasonably argue that when the measurement proved to be imprecise false-positive cases were removed while possible false-negative cases were ignored.

For these reasons, it is preferable to follow the suggestions by the Committee for Proprietary Medicinal Products (CPMP), which require a measurement by cardiologists with an appropriate quality control. As an example, the

Department of Cardiological Sciences at St George's Hospital Medical School in London developed a standard of practice involving digital on-screen measurements of electrocardiograms with simultaneously recorded 12 leads. In each electrocardiogram, five suitable cardiac cycles are identified and the QT interval is measured in all leads of all five cycles by two or three (or even four, if the highest precision is required) mutually independent cardiologists. The measurement of the QT interval includes morphological classification of repolarization patterns and categories of T/U amalgamation. Those electrocardiographic leads are identified for which the observers differed by more than an agreed limit (e.g., 25 ms) or for which they disagreed on the morphological T/U classification (this usually concerns approximately 20–30% of all leads). These leads are returned to the same cardiologists for second blind and independent measurement and if a disagreement still exists, the measurement and morphological classification is reconciled by two of the most senior cardiologists of the Department (this usually concerns approximately 5–10% of all leads). In each lead, the QT intervals measured in separate cardiac cycles are averaged and lead-specific QT interval durations are obtained. From the QT interval durations in all leads that were found measurable, either the median (and/or maximum) QT interval is derived and used to express the QT duration in the given electrocardiogram. These QT interval values are corrected for heart rate using the mean of all sinus rhythm P–P intervals that appear in the complete recording (usually 10 s). Recordings that contain arrhythmia are generally discarded; although some part of the recording may be usable, the data may be too difficult to interpret.

Rate correction

A change in heart rate may occur due to the direct effects of the compound on the sinus node, indirect therapeutic effects (e.g., anti-inflammatory effects when studying an antibiotic), autonomic conditioning of the subjects during the study, as well as a simple psychological placebo effect. The QT interval is not constant and varies inversely with the heart rate. Therefore, when assessing or comparing whether or not the intrinsic duration of the QT interval has been altered by a pathological process or a drug, the QT interval must be corrected for heart rate.

Some advocate measuring the RR interval preceding the QT interval for rate correction. Unfortunately, this simple approach is incorrect. The QT interval does not depend on the immediately preceding RR interval but on the underlying heart rate. The adaptation to the changes in heart rate is gradual with 90% of the adaptation achieved in approximately 2 min after a sudden heart rate change. Thus, the average RR interval representing the ambient heart rate of the whole ECG sample needs to be measured. Moreover, ECGs recorded while heart rate is accelerating or decelerating are unsuitable for the assessment of rate corrected QT interval. Because of the hysteresis lag of QT/RR adaptation, the synchrony between the QT and RR intervals is lost during such recordings.

QT/RR hysteresis is important not only for proper heart rate correction of the QT interval. When the QT interval is measured during or just after a change in heart rate, the heart rate to use in the analysis of that QT interval is not defined (Fig. 3.12). More precisely, when a recording is made while heart rate is accelerating, the simultaneously recorded QT and RR intervals do not belong together because the QT interval did not yet have the time to adapt to the new level of heart rate. Artefactual QTc interval increase will result. Likewise, recordings taken while heart rate is decelerating leads to artefactual QTc interval shortening. The QT/RR hysteresis has also serious implications for the so-called "bin method" which aims at avoiding heart rate correction by comparing QT intervals that occur at the same heart rate, standardly implemented as QT intervals following the same duration of an RR interval. Such an implementation of the bin method leads to gross and substantial errors since respiratory arrhythmia and other short-term variations in RR interval duration make one single RR interval a very poor expression of the underlying heart rate (Fig. 3.13).

Of all the formulas used in the past, the most commonly used are Bazett's square-root formula ($QTc = QT/RR^{1/2}$) and Fridericia's cube-root formula ($QTc = QT/RR^{1/3}$). Between the two, Bazett's formula is more commonly used and most reported normal values are given using Bazett's formula, mainly because of its simplicity (most simple calculators have a function for a square root but not for a cube-root computation which gives a practical "advantage" to Bazett's over Fridericia's correction). Some argue that

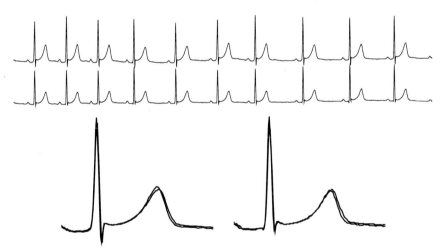

Fig. 3.12 Example of QT/RR hysteresis. The top panel shows leads V4 and V6 of a 10 sec electrocardiogram recorded while heart rate was decelerating (consecutive RR intervals of 768, 764, 858, 982, 984, 904, 1144, 1120, and 1056 ms). The bottom part of the figure shows superimposition of the QRS-T complexes following the shortest (764 ms) and longest (1144 ms) RR intervals. Despite the substantial difference in RR intervals, the QT interval is constant at 376 ms. Using the Bazett correction, the QTc interval ranges from 352 ms to 430 ms in the tracing demonstrating that to use the previous RR interval for the QT interval correction is bizarrely wrong.

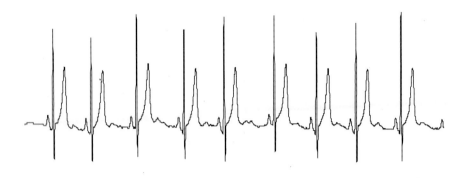

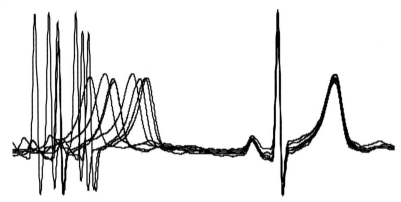

Fig. 3.13 One of the problems with the "bin method" if ignoring QT/RR hysteresis. The top panel shows a 10 sec 1 lead recording in which the RR intervals are visibly very variable. The bottom panel shows superimposition of all 8 RR intervals aligned by the R peak of the second QRS complex. Although the QT intervals in the recordings are preceded by very different RR intervals, they are literally identical. Incorporation of these identical QT intervals into the very different bins of the different RR intervals leads to gross inaccuracies. (Courtesy of Dr V N Batchvarov.)

Fridericia's correction is preferred because it is more accurate at the extremes of physiological heart rate [23,26], whereas Bazett's formula overcorrects the measured QT interval*. It is now well recognized that Bazett's formula is the least accurate and thus the least appropriate.

* The terms undercorrection and overcorrection of the QT interval are frequently used without much insight. It seems therefore appropriate to suggest the following terminology: uncorrected QT interval increases with increasing values of RR interval and thus, the correlation between uncorrected QT interval and RR interval is positive as is the slope of the QT/RR regression. The goal of a correction formula is to produce QTc values that are uncorrelated with RR intervals and thus have the slope of QTc/RR regression 0. Hence, in essence, a correction formula should tilt (as well as straighten) the QT/RR pattern so that the QTc/RR relationship is a flat line. Those formulae that tilt the QT/RR pattern too much (and

Surprisingly, while the problems of the Bazett correction with drugs that change heart rate are well known and are frequently discussed when a drug that accelerates heart rate leads to artificial QTc (Bazett) prolongation, some researchers and cardiologists seem not to be fully aware of the opposite possibility. For instance, Bazett correction leads to substantial and highly significant (and artificial) shortening of the QTc interval on beta-blockers [27]. Thus, the Bazett correction may easily mask a substantial QT interval prolongation and signs of proarrhythmic toxicity with drugs that slow heart rate. Moreover, since bradycardia is one of the predisposing factors of TdP initiation, this potential oversight may have serious consequences.

There are many formulas that have been proposed to replace the most frequently used Bazett formula to correct the QT interval (QTc) for the biophysical effect of heart rate (Table 3.1) [28–51]. Unfortunately, no one equation stands out as the best overall and there is no scientific evidence to prefer one formula to the others. Each of the new proposals was based on an assumption that a "physiological" pattern of the QT/RR relationship exists which might be approximated by pooling the data of different subjects. In this assumption, it is overlooked that if a universal "physiological" pattern of QT/RR relationship existed, the various studies reporting different heart rate correction formulas would not have led to such conflicting results.

Some of these formulas originate from epidemiological studies, which are often performed retrospectively and will need to be validated prospectively before they are applied to a general population that may be characteristically different from the original population. Furthermore, a formula that best fits the QT vs. RR data in a large population does not necessarily optimally describe the relation in a given individual and vice versa. Thus, no single rate correction formula is likely to be universally applicable. When assessing the proarrhythmic effect of a drug, the rate-corrected QTc interval should be independent of heart rate because the comparison of QTc values before and after the introduction of a drug might otherwise be influenced by changes in heart rate. A false-positive or false-negative conclusion might be made depending on the change of heart rate with the treatment and the overcorrection or undercorrrection implicit with the formula used to derive the QTc.

thus lead to a negative correlation between QTc and RR and to a negative QTc/RR slope) **overcorrect** while those formulae that tilt the QT/RR too little (and thus lead to a still positive correlation between QTc and RR and to a positive QTc/RR slope) **undercorrect**.

As an example: in a study of 50 healthy volunteers, the individual correlation coefficients between QTc (Bazett) and RR intervals ranged between −0.877 and −0.089 (that it is Bazett's formula overcorrected in each case) while the individual correlation coefficients between QTc (Fridericia) and RR intervals ranged between −0.598 and +0.686 with 12 cases of negative correlation (overcorrection) and 38 cases of positive correlation (undercorrection). Only in 11 cases of the 50 subjects was the correlation coefficient between QTc (Fridericia) and RR intervals within the limits of −0.1 and +0.1 which, although still not entirely precise, might perhaps be accepted as a practically reasonable correction. (There was only 1 such case with Bazett's formula.)

Table 3.1 Various formulae used to correct QT interval for heart rate.

Formula	Mathematical formula	Comments
Bazet [28]	$QT/RR^{0.5}$	Most commonly used but inaccurate at extreme of heart rates
Fridericia [29]	$QT/RR^{0.333}$	
Mayeda [30]	$QT/RR^{0.604}$	Adult cohort without heart disease
Kawataki [31]	$QT/RR^{0.25}$	
Yoshinaga [32]	$QT/RR^{0.31}$	Children
Boudoulas [33]	$QT/RR^{0.398}$	Patients undergoing minimally stressful diagnostic tests
Ashman [34]	$QT/\log(10RR + 0.07)$	Children (0–14 year) included. A reference RR of 930 ms used
Adams [35]	$QT + 0.1464(1\text{-}RR)$ (all subject)	Gender-based formula
	$QT + 0.1536(1\text{-}RR)$ (male)	
	$QT + 0.1259(1\text{-}RR)$ (female)	
Ljung [36]	$QT + 0.2(1\text{-}RR)$	Adults with hypocalcaemia
Schlamowitz [37]	$QT + 0.205(1\text{-}RR)$	Healthy soldiers at rest and after exercise
Simonson [38]	$QT + 0.14(1\text{-}RR)$	Healthy subjects
Framingham [39]	$QT + 0.154(1\text{-}RR)$	Population-based study (noncardiac)
Akhras & Rickards [40,41]	$QT + 1.87(HR\text{-}60)$	Mixture of patients undergoing treadmill exercise to evaluate QT-RR relationship (patients taking beta-blockers, patients with complete heart block exercised with fixed ventricular pacing at 70 bpm & patients with atrial pacing/stress testing)
Hodges [42]	$QT + 1.75(HR\text{-}60)$	Healthy subjects
Kligfield [43]	$QT + 1.32(HR\text{-}60)$	
Wohlfart [44]	$QT + 1.23(HR\text{-}60)$	
Karjalainen [45]	values in a published table	
Rautaharju [46,47]	$QT/(1 + 1.41 \times 10^{-5}QT(60\text{-}HR))$ (male) $QT/(1 + 1.54 \times 10^{-5}QT(60\text{-}HR))$ (female)	Men only, formula intended for hear rate 60–100 bpm. Population-based study
Kovacs [48]	$QTc = QT\text{-}0.656/(1 + 0.01\times HR) + 0.41$	
Arrowood [49]	$QTc = QT + 0.304\text{-}0.492xe^{(-0.008 \times HR)}$	
Sarma [50]	$QTc = QT\text{-}0.0149\text{-}0.664 \times e^{-2.7\times HR}$	Mixture of healthy subjects undergoing bicycle exercise and patients with VVI pacing
Lecocq [51]	$QTc = QT\text{-}0.017\text{-}0.676 \times e^{-3.7\times HR}$	

The use of a universal heart rate correction formula in drug studies is based on the assumption that the mathematical curve corresponding to the formula provides a reasonable fit not only to the pooled drug-free data of the whole group but also to the drug-free data of each individual participant. Such an assumption must be satisfied in order to obtain QTc interval values that are truly independent of heart rate; QTc interval data need to be independent of heart rate because the comparison of on- and off-treatment recordings that might otherwise be influenced by changes in heart rate and both false-positive and false-negative conclusions might be reached (dependence on the change of heart rate on-treatment and on the overcorrection or under-correction of the formula used). If any of these assumptions are not satisfied, a drug that changes heart rate (directly or indirectly) might be artificially reported to change (or not change) the QTc interval purely due to the over- or undercorrection by an inappropriate formula.

Previously proposed universal heart rate correction formulas have been derived from population data and the large differences between these formulas suggest that the QT/RR relationship has not been found reproducible from study to study. It is therefore unreasonable to expect that a general formula selected from those previously published will satisfy the drug-free QT/RR relationship for the data of a given study. For this reason, it has been proposed that the drug-free data of each new study might be used to develop a heart rate correction formula that will fit the need of the particular data in hand. Linear as well as nonlinear regression modelling of the QT and RR interval data points have been proposed. Indeed, a log/log linear formula $QT = \beta \times RR^{\alpha}$ leads to a very simple heart rate correction in the form of $QTc = QT/RR^{\alpha}$. Thus, all the drug-free QT/RR interval data of a given study might be subjected to log/log linear modelling and a simple study-specific correction formula derived from the model. Thus, the exact form of the formula clearly depends on the distribution of the drug-free data. Although it has been reported that the formula $QTc = RR^{0.37}$ satisfies different data sets [52,53], this observation has not been reproduced in more recent investigations [54].

When a sufficient number of baseline (e.g., drug free) electrocardiograms are available from each of the investigated subjects, the individualized heart rate correction formula should also reflect the curvature of the subject specific QT/RR relationship. Experience shows that by ignoring the curvature, errors of up to 10 or 15 ms might be introduced. In particular, the log/log linear formula $QTc = QT/RR^{\alpha}$ that gained some popularity because of its mathematical simplicity is frequently a poor possibility. More precise heart rate correction is achieved with other nonlinear regression models that need to be individually selected from a spectrum of different QT/RR curvatures.

The concept of pooled regression analysis improves the heart rate correction by ensuring that in the pooled data of a study, the QTc intervals are statistically independent of the RR intervals. However, the concept of the pooled regression is based on the assumption that the QT/RR relationship is equivalent in all subjects of the study (the same assumption is made when applying any pooled formula, irrespective of whether it is universal or data-specific).

Only recently, has it been possible to record frequent serial 12-lead electrocardiograms in the same individual using a 12-lead Holter recorder. Studies utilizing this technology have suggested that the concept of a "physiological" QT/RR relationship that is identical in every healthy individual, is inherently flawed. A study conducted at St George's Hospital Medical School in London [55] recorded serial 12-lead electrocardiograms in 75 healthy volunteers. Each of the subjects underwent repeated ambulatory 12-lead monitoring using the SEER MC recorders by GE Marquette Medical Systems. The recorders were programmed to obtain a 10-s 12-lead electrocardiogram every 30 s for the whole duration of a nominal 24-h period. In each subject, the recording was repeated 1 day, 1 week, and 1 month later. In total, four sets of 24-h data were obtained in each individual. The separate 12-lead electrocardiograms were subsequently processed using the QT Guard system by GE Marquette to obtain an automatic reading of heart rate and of the median duration of QT interval of all the 12 ECG leads (that is, the median value of all measurable leads was used). While the automatic measurement of the QT interval in 12-lead electrocardiograms is potentially problematic, this study utilized automatic readings purely because of the sheer volume of electrocardiograms to be processed. The data from this study showed that while the QT/RR pattern was stable in each individual, it differed substantially from subject to subject (Fig. 3.14). In addition to the visual observations, a nonlinear regression $QT = \beta \times RR^{\alpha}$ was obtained between the QT and RR interval data points of each 24-h recording. The values of the parameters β (slope) and α (curvature) of individual subjects differed considerably but the regression parameters β and α remained relatively stable in each individual. Thus, the QT/RR relationship exhibits a high intrasubject stability with a high intersubject variability. This study shows that even in a population of healthy subjects, no single mathematical formula can be obtained which will describe the QT/RR relationship satisfactorily in all individuals.

Moreover, the curvatures of QT/RR relationship of separate individuals are frequently on average flatter (and occasionally steeper) than their pooled composition (that is, the average of individual slopes α is significantly lower than the slope $\bar{\alpha}$ of the pooled regression). This suggests that even a formula derived from a pooled regression of all drug-free data of the study might systematically over- or undercorrect when applied to separate individuals. For these reasons, a drug-free pattern of the QT/RR relationship should be examined in each participant when assessing the proarrhythmic potential of a drug so that no methodological inaccuracy in heart rate correction is introduced. It seems that only in this way, is meaningful outlier analysis possible.

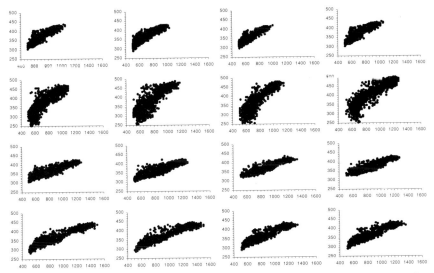

Fig. 3.14 Forms of QT/RR relationship in 4 different healthy subjects. The four rows correspond to 4 different healthy subjects in whom the recordings have been repeated (from left to right) at day 0, 1, 7 and 30. Note the marked intersubject differences and intrasubject stability. (The horizontal axes show RR intervals and the vertical axes corresponding QT intervals in milliseconds.)

QT parameters for assessment of proarrhythmias

In addition to the simple QT interval assessed in a particular ECG lead, many other methods have been proposed to assess the repolarization abnormality. The Committee for Proprietary Medicinal Products (CPMP) suggested that maximum QTc interval, maximum change from baseline (ΔQTc) and QT dispersion should be assessed during drug developmental stage to examine any potential proarrhythmic effect. In addition to these simple derived parameters, novel techniques to categorize and quantify the morphological change of the T wave are presently under active development. Although only limited experience exists at present, it seems likely that these new methods will not only provide further information on repolarization abnormality induced by drug or disease but perhaps supersede the present assessment that is based solely on the QT interval measurement.

Maximum QTc interval

Generally, QT prolongation is considered when the QTc interval is greater than 440 ms (men) and 460 ms (women) [19], using the Bazett's formula (Table 3.2). The CPMP suggested the upper limit of normal QTc interval for adult males be 450 ms and adult female be 470 ms [56]. The severity of proarrhythmia at a given QT interval varies from drug to drug and from patient to patient. Although the QT interval is frequently viewed as a

Table 3.2 Normal values of QTc interval (Bazett's correction).

	QTc interval		
Moss [52]	*Normal*	*Borderline*	*Prolonged (top 1%)*
Adult men	<430 ms	430–450 ms	>450 ms
Adult women	<450 ms	450–470 ms	>470 ms
Children (1–15 year)	<440 ms	440–460 ms	>460 ms
Levels			
Adult men	450 ms (upper limit)		
Adult women	470 ms (upper limit)	CPMP [58]	
Concern of drug-effect	500 ms		

surrogate marker of the arrhythmogenic potential of a drug, the extent of QT prolongation and risk of TdP with a given drug may not be linearly related to the dose or plasma level of the drug because patient-specific and metabolic factors are also important (e.g., gender, electrolyte level, etc.). Furthermore, except in the case of congenital long QT syndrome, there have been very few data to quantify the magnitude of arrhythmic risk assessment with particular values of QT prolongation, especially with drug-induced QT prolongation. In drug-induced long QT syndrome, there appears to be no linear relationship between the degree of drug induced QT prolongation and the likelihood of the development of TdP [57]. TdP can sometimes occur without any prolongation of the QT interval, although this is unusual.

In the case of congenital LQTS, data from the LQTS Registry showed that the risk of malignant ventricular arrhythmias is exponentially related to the length of QTc interval [19]. In this registry, 1496 enrolled subjects (probands, affected and unaffected family members), the hazard ratio for cardiac events (arrhythmic syncope or probable long QT syndrome-related death) was 1.052^x (95% C.I. 1.017–1.088) where "x" is the per 0.01 second unit increase in QTc beyond 0.45 [19]. Thus, a patient with QTc of 0.60 s would have a 2.76-fold increase risk of a cardiac event at follow-up compared to a subject with QTc of 0.40 s (hazard ratio = 2.76). However, the confidence interval of 1.017–1.088 is rather large when used in the exponential formula (in the given example, the confidence interval of the hazard ratio ranges from 1.40 to 5.40). Moreover the stability of the form of the proposed statistical model was not (and could hardly have been) tested. That is, it is not obvious whether the same model applies to "small" and "large" QT interval prolongation. Therefore, this analysis of the congenital LQTS Registry does not actually address the question whether a tiny QT interval prolongation by only a few milliseconds carries any measurable proarrhythmic risk at all.

In drug-induced QT prolongation, no such relationship is known or has ever been proposed. A MEDLINE search of the English-language literature for the period of 1980 through 1992, on proarrhythmia (TdP, polymorphic ventricular tachycardia, atypical ventricular tachycardia, and drug-induced ventricular tachycardia) by cardiac drugs known to prolong QT interval showed that, among the 332 patients with proarrhythmia, while only 25% of the patients had baseline QTc $\geq$ 470 ms, 90% of them had QTc $\geq$ 500 ms when they developed arrhythmias [58]. Thus, the CPMP proposed that a maximal QTc value of over 500 ms should cause concern about the potential for drug-induced TdP [57]. Bonate and Russell estimated that the false positive rate for maximal QTc interval ($>$450 ms) was about 7% [59]. Although these values seem reasonable, the false-positive rate for borderline prolongation (431–450 ms) is about 7–28% [59]. Thus, the guideline proposed by the CPMP for borderline cases is potentially erroneous in identifying marginally prolonged QTc interval. Woosley suggested that the number of ECGs/subject could be increased to improve the power of the ECG to detect minor pharmacological effects on the QT interval [60].

It has been suggested that in some patients, postpause accentuation of the U wave, if present, may be a better predictor of TdP than the duration of QTc interval [61], particularly with drug-associated TdP. When an ectopic beat or brief tachycardia is followed by a pause, it is therefore important to examine the QT interval and T/U wave morphology in the postextrasystolic sinus beat [61] as drug-induced changes in the T wave morphology and/or the occurrence of a U wave are probably as significant as QT prolongation itself.

QT dispersion

When originally proposed, QT dispersion (the range, i.e., maximum—minimum QT interval in different leads of the 12-lead surface ECG) was considered to be an indirect measure of spatial heterogeneity of repolarization and may be useful in assessing drug efficacy and safety. In one initial study, patients who received a class Ia antiarrhythmic drug and developed TdP had significantly increased precordial QT interval dispersion [62]. In contrast, patients receiving amiodarone or class Ia antiarrhythmics (principally quinidine) without TdP, did not have increased precordial QT dispersion although the QT interval was noticeably prolonged and not different between both groups [63]. Thus, it was believed that QT dispersion addressed the spatial heterogeneity or dispersion of the ventricular repolarization process and may be required for the initiation of TdP.

Amiodarone has been reported to decrease [63–65] or not to alter [62,66,67], QT dispersion. It is known that amiodarone can be administered relatively safely in patients who had experienced TdP during antiarrhythmic therapy with other drugs and this effect is paralleled by a decrease of QT dispersion. Cui *et al.* measured the QTc interval and QT dispersion in two groups of patients with cardiac arrhythmias and intraventricular conduction delays before and after treatment with amiodarone and with quinidine [63]. While both amiodarone and quinidine increased the QTc interval, amiodarone reduced QT dispersion by 40% (90 ± 17 to 54 ± 13, $P < 0.001$), whereas quinidine increased QT dispersion by 18% (80 ± 14 to 94 ± 19 ms, $P < 0.001$). Similarly, in another study by the same authors, amiodarone, sematilide, and sotalol all significantly prolonged the QTc interval but only amiodarone significantly reduced QT dispersion (79 ± 13 to 49 ± 14 ms; $P < 0.001$) [64].

In contrast, other QT prolonging antiarrhythmics such as quinidine, sotalol, sematilide, almokalant have all been reported to increse the QT dispersion [64,68,69]. In one study of patients treated for chronic atrial fibrillation, quinidine induced TdP in 3/25 patients[12%] who reverted to sinus rhythm. In these patients, QT dispersion increased by >50% of the baseline value [68]. Similarly, Houltz et al. [69] studied the effect of class III drug almokalant (a pure I_{Kr} blocker) on 100 patients with atrial fibrillation and 62 patients in sinus rhythm. Six of the patients with atrial fibrillation developed TdP during almokalant infusion. The QT dispersion in both the precordial and limb leads in these patients was significantly greater than in those who did not develop TdP.

The data on the effect of sotalol on QT dispersion is controversial. While some workers reported increased QT dispersion with sotalol [64], others did not [70,71]. Hohnloser et al. [71] studied the effect of sotalol in 50 patients treated for ventricular tachycardia/fibrillation. QT dispersion was significantly decreased in 19 patients who responded to sotalol (from 61 ± 18 to 45 ± 16 ms, $P < 0.01$), not changed in 20 patients who did not respond to the therapy (from 58 ± 23 to 53 ± 13 ms, $p = N.S$), and was significantly increased in 11 patients who developed TdP as a result of sotalol therapy (from 56 ± 26 to 85 ± 34 ms, $P < 0.05$).

Despite these initial results, the practical use of QT dispersion for the prediction of TdP is limited not only because of measurement difficulties, lack of standardized methodology and established normal limits, and by poor and inconsistent interobserver and intraobserver reproducibility [18,72] but also, perhaps more importantly, by a poorly defined electrocardiographic concept and simplistic definition of the technology. Malik and Batchvarov reviewed 51 studies involving 8455 healthy controls and the mean value of normal QT dispersion among these studies was reported to be between 30 and 50 ms and the weighted mean was 33.4 ± 20.3 ms [73]. While different cardiac conditions, including patients with hypertrophic cardiomyopathy, dilated cardiomyopathy, left ventricular hypertrophy, congenital long QT syndrome, present with different degrees of increased QT dispersion [73], the prognostic value of QT dispersion in predicting ventricular tachyarrhythmias or sudden death in other clinical settings remains controversial [74–76]. For this reason, whilst the lack of increased QT dispersion is not reassuring, only extreme values of QT dispersion or an extreme increase of QT dispersion on therapy may be considered as an indication of a gross repolarization abnormality and should then be treated as an indicator of high risk. Such extreme values will almost certainly be found only in cases of gross T wave morpological abnormalities which are warning signs in their own right. Thus, it is highly questionable whether QT dispersion assessment actually adds anything to the estimation of proarrhythmic danger: most probably, it does not.

Still the present document of the CPMP suggests that QT dispersion of >100 ms and/or a change of >100% from baseline be considered as associated with an increased risk of arrhythmias [77–79]. While an increase of QT dispersion above 100 ms will almost certainly indicate a marked repolarization abnormality, and an increase by >100% from baseline (e.g., from 17 ms to 35 ms) can be very easily obtained purely by measurement inaccuracy and seems to have no practical value. Thus, this particular recommendation of CPMP has to be interpreted with caution.

Repolarization morphology

No studies presently exist evaluating more focused descriptors of T wave loop abnormalities and/or repolarization sequence disturbances in patients with drug-induced TdP. Newer and more detailed methods of describing ventricular repolarization have been introduced [80], and may potentially be sensitive in distinguishing "good" from "bad" QT prolonging drugs and the risk of TdP. T wave morphology can also be used to assess abnormal rather than delayed repolarization and may give an early indication of the pro-arrhythmic risk. Various QT methods of assessing repolarization have also been proposed and may overcome the shortfalls of QTc interval.

Maximum change from baseline (ΔQTc)

Apart from the maximum QTc interval, the current guidelines proposed by the CPMP have also suggested that the individual maximum QTc change relative to drug-free baseline (ΔQTc) should also be measured. The major problem with this method is that unless both baseline and postdrug measurements are made under the same conditions, it is difficult to determine whether the value obtained is a result of the drug intervention or due to inherent variability of the QTc interval over time or to other confounding factors such as posture and circadian changes. This method also fails to take account of "regression towards the mean". A QTc interval that is relatively long for a given individual is more likely to be followed, in a random sampling of that individual, by a shorter rather than a longer interval and an individual whose baseline QTc interval is below the mean will tend to have a longer subsequent QT [59]. Thus, multiple measurements are crucial when determining the normal range for ΔQTc. Morganroth *et al.* observed that using Holter monitoring that in normal male subjects aged between 25 and 53 years, the intrasubject QTc variability over 24 h is 76 ± 19 ms [81]. However, since these data were based on Bazett's correction, they are certainly polluted by the known circadian pattern of heart rate, which makes this observation at best problematic. The circadian variation of QTc interval has also been reported by others using 12-lead ECGs and Holter recordings [82–84]. Pratt *et al.* found that normal subjects and patients with cardiovascular disease had a large range of QTc values (average QTc fluctuation: 66 ± 15 ms) [85]. However, the same limitation due to the use of Bazett's formula applies. A MEDLINE search on QT prolonging cardiac drug-induced arrhythmia (TdP, polymorphic ventricular tachycardia, atypical ventricular tachycardia, and drug-induced ventricular tachycardia) by Makkar *et al.* showed that most of the patients with drug-induced proarrhythmias had a very similar maximum QTc interval while receiving the cardiac drugs (580–600 ± 60–70 ms) [58], irrespective of their baseline QTc interval. However, the ΔQTc in these patients were very different. In patients with the longest baseline QTc interval (≥470 ms), the mean ΔQTc was 70 ± 80 ms whereas in patients with the shortest baseline QTc interval (≤410 ms), the ΔQTc can be as much as 200 ± 50 ms. The circadian rhythmicity of QTc interval is likely to be related to autonomic modulation of the ventricular repolarization, since diabetic patients with proven autonomic neuropathy or denervated transplanted human heart had no circadian variation of the QTc interval [84,86]. Morganroth suggested that a threshold of ΔQTc >75 ms should therefore be considered clinically abnormal [81]. Using this threshold of ΔQTc of 75 ms, the sensitivity and specificity of identifying patients at risk of TdP are 70% and 89%, respectively [87]. The CPMP proposed that a ΔQTc interval between 30 and 60 ms is likely to represent a drug effect, and changes of greater than 60 ms should raise concerns about the potential proarrhythmic risk for a new drug (Table 3.3) [56]. The false-positive rate for ΔQTc > 60 ms is estimated to be about 1% and for borderline ΔQTc (30–60 ms) is believed to be 1–12% [59].

Time-averaged QTc intervals

In drug-induced QT prolongation, the time-averaged QTc interval may also be used [46]. Multiple measurements on each subject are collapsed into a single mean or summary value, removing the influence of time, with each subject's predose QTc interval as a covariate. This approach may be used if there is no clear concentration–effect relationship and has the advantage that it is easy to calculate and interpret. For instance, Pratt *et al.* used this method and showed that the averaged QTc interval after 5 days of twice-daily dosing of terfenadine 60 mg in healthy, normal subjects was 409 ms compared to 403 ms at baseline ($P < 0.03$) [85]. However, there are limitations with this method. For instance, it assumes that intrasubject variation is entirely due to random noise, which may not be the case, since QTc intervals are subject to circadian variation. Therefore, the random noise assumption is violated if the data are collected during both day and night [59]. Furthermore, since the QTc

---

QTc interval:
- Individual increases <30 ms unlikely to raise concerns
- 30–60 ms increases likely to be a drug effect
- >60 ms increases raise concerns of possible TdP or QT
- Absolute QTc (Bazett's or Fridericia) >500 ms raise concerns of possible TdP

Table 3.3 Guidelines and prolongation of QTc interval.

interval is affected by drug concentration, averaging the QTc interval will underestimate the magnitude of true maximal QTc dose/concentration–response relationship and decrease the power to detect significant QTc prolongation [59].

Area under the QTc interval–time curve

To overcome the problem of temporal variation of QTc interval, the area under the QTc interval–time curve method may be potentially more useful. With this method, repeated-measurements are collapsed into a univariate summary measure that represents an integrated effect over time and is more stable to random fluctuations [59]. It is important that both baseline and postdose data are collected at the same time points for parallel comparison and that a sufficient number of data points are derived for each subject to compute the area under curve [59]. The drawback with this method is the uncertainly over the preference on the point of reference, none of which is perfect. In the method that uses 0 ms as the reference point, a minor drug effect may not be detectable. On the other hand, if the integration is performed around the baseline QTc interval, it is uncertain whether all areas get treated as positive areas contributing to total area under the curve, or areas below the baseline be treated as negative area subtracting from the positive area under the curve [59].

QT/RR relationship (QT dynamicity)

As discussed previously, the QT interval is influenced by autonomic tone and exhibits a circadian rhythmicity. Thus, it is suggested that the QT/RR dynamic relationship or QT dynamicity (i.e., beat-to-beat changes of the QT interval vs. beat-to-beat changes of the RR intervals over the 24-h period) as measured on Holter recording will provide more information on the dynamic heterogeneity of ventricular repolarization and sympathovagal imbalance, and hence will perform better as a predictor of arrhythmic risk [23].

However, the technique has not been widely adopted and has many technical limitations. For instance, the large number of complexes analyzed requires an automatic approach which is problematic. The reduced number of leads available for analysis and the frequent presence of noise in the recording make data less reliable [23].

There is not as yet an agreed algorithmic method for calculating QT dynamicity. Most studies have so far utilized the correlation of the slope of QT/RR dynamic relationship from 24-h Holter recording. Others investigators use power spectral analysis. In patients with QT prolonging drugs, an increased slope of QT/RR relationship has been reported [23]. Kadish *et al.* examined the QT dynamicity and the rate dependence of the QT interval with exercise in patients with previous TdP due to class Ia antiarrhythmic drugs (quinidine, procainamide and disopyramide) in the absence of these drugs [88]. They showed that the response of QT interval to exercise is abnormal in patients with TdP compared with those without TdP while taking the same type of drugs. The degree of QT shortening with exercise was less in the TdP group compared with controls, despite a similar decrease in cycle length in both groups. Thus, the QTc interval was paradoxically prolonged in those patients with TdP.

Sharma and colleagues suggested that the information obtained from QT dynamicity could also be used to assess the reverse-use-dependency of a QT-prolonging drug [83]. The steeper the slope of the regression curve of QT/RR dynamic relationship (termed reverse-use-dependency index by the authors), the higher the reverse-use-dependency of the drug (Fig. 3.15). This, and other observations, highlight the little considered notion that the relationship of the QT interval to heart rate, and therefore heart rate correction formulas, may be different in the control and drug treatment conditions.

Of note, the QT intervals measurement obtained from 24-h Holter recording also provides information on the effect of a drug on the circadian pattern of heart rate and QT dynamicity. For instance, sotalol abolished the circadian variation of heart rate while preserving the circadian rhythmicity of QT (and QTc) interval [82]. In contrast, amiodarone abolished QT and QTc circadian variability but preserved the RR variability [89]. Thus, in contrast to sotalol, amiodarone suppressed the direct autonomic modulation of ventricular repolarization. The inference from this observation is that the antiarrhythmic action and low incidence of proarrhythmia by amiodarone is probably mediated by a combination of factors including continuous bradycardia and

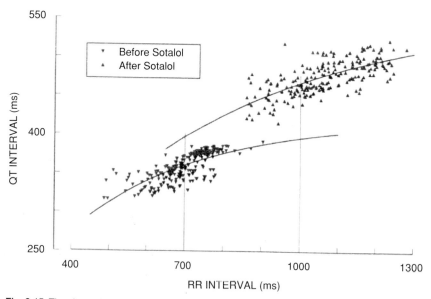

Fig. 3.15 The slope of the QT/RR regression line (QT dynamicity or reverse-use-dependency) increased after the introduction of sotalol (adapted from [85]).

the uniform prolongation of myocardial repolarization with reduced temporal (and spatial) variabilities [89].

Thus, it seems likely that QT dynamicity may offer additional information on the drug-induced QT effect that could not be obtained by other means. However, all the present data need to be interpreted with caution since technical settings differ from study to study and details of the technologies, that may be primarily responsible for the character of observations made, are frequently not reported.

References

1 Surawicz B, Knoebel S. Long QT: good, bad or indifferent? *J Am Coll Cardiol* 1984; 4: 398–413.

2 Lepeschkin E, Surawicz B. The measurement of the Q-T interval of the electrocardiogram. *Circulation* 1952; 6: 378–88.

3 Kautzner J, Yi G, Kishore R *et al*. Interobserver reproducibility of QT interval measurement and QT dispersion in patients after acute myocardial infarction. *Ann Noninvas Electrocardiol* 1996; 1: 363–74.

4 Watanabe Y. Purkinje repolarization as a possible cause of the U wave in the electrocardiogram. *Circulation* 1975; 51: 1030–7.

5 Lepeschkin E. Physiologic basis of the U wave. In: Schlant, RC, Hurst, JW, eds. *Advances in Electrocardiography*. Grune & Stratton, New York and London 1972, 431–47.

6 Yan G-Y, Antzelevich C. Cellular Basis for the Normal T wave and the electrocardiographic manifestations of the long QT syndrome. *Circulation* 1998; 98: 1928–36.

7 Benardeau A, Weissenburger J, Hondeghem L *et al*. Effects of the T-type Ca (2+) channel blocker mibefradil on repolarization of guinea pig, rabbit, dog, monkey, and human cardiac tissue. *J Pharmacol Exp Ther* 2000; 292: 561–75.

8 Murray A, McLaughlin NB, Bourke JP, Doig JC, Furniss SS, Campbell RWP. Errors in manual measurement of QT interval. *Br Heart J* 1994; 71: 386–90.

9 Ahnve S, Gilpin E, Madsen Eb Froelicher V, Henning H, Ross J. Prognostic importance of QTc interval at discharge after myocardial infarction: a multicentre study of 865 patients. *Am Heart J* 1984; 108: 395–400.

10 Juul-Moller S. Corrected QT interval during one year follow-up after an acute myocardial infarction. *Eur Heart J* 1986; 7: 299–304.

11 Wheelan K, Mukharji J, Rude RE *et al*. Sudden death and its relation to QT prolongation after myocardial infarction: two-year follow-up. *Am J Cardiol* 1986; 57: 745–50.

12 Schamroth L. *An Introduction to Electrocardiography*, 6th edn. Pitman Medical, Tunbridge Well 1978.

13 Cowan JC, Yusoff K, Moore M *et al*. Importance of lead selection in the QT interval measurement. *Am J Cardiol* 1988; 61: 83–7.

14 Malik M, Batchvarov VN. Measurement, interpretation and clinical potential of QT dispersion. *J Am Coll Cardiol* 2000; 36: 1749–66.

15 Murray A, McLaughlin NB, Bourke JP, Doig JC, Furniss SS, Campbell RW. Errors in manual measurement of QT intervals. *B Heart J* 1994; 71: 386–90.

16 Ahnve S. Errors in the visual determination of corrected QT (QTc) interval during acute myocardial infarction. *J Am Coll Cardiol* 1985; 5: 699–702.

17 Malik M, Bradford A. Human precision of operating a digitizing board: implications for electrocardiogram measurements. *PACE* 1998; 21: 1656–62.

18 Savelieva I, Yi G, Guo X, Hnatkova K, Malik M Agreement and reproducibility of automatic versus manual measurement of QT interval and QT dispersion. *Am J Cardiol* 1998; 81 (4): 471–7.

19 Childers R. Risk assessment: the 12-lead electrocardiogram. In: Malik M. (ed) *Risk of Arrhythmia and Sudden Death*. BMJ Books, London 2001, pp. 65–97.

20 McLaughlin NB, Campbell RWF, Murray A. Accuracy of four automatic QT measurement techniques in cardiac patients and healthy subjects. *Heart* 1996; 76: 422–6.

21 McLaughlin NB, Campbell RWF, Murray A. Comparison of automatic QT measurement techniques in the normal 12 lead electrocardiogram. *Br Heart J* 1995; 74: 84–9.

22 Xue Q, Reddy S. Algorithms for computerized QT analysis. *J Electrocardiol* 1998; 30: 181–6.

23 Funck-Brentano C, Jaillon P. Rate-corrected QT interval: techniques and limitation. *Am J Cardiol* 1993; 72: 17B–22B.

24 Maison-Blanche P, Coumel P. Changes in repolarization dynamicity and the assessment of the arrhythmic risk. *Pacing Clin Electrophysiol* 1997; 20 (10 Part 2): 2614–24.

25 Garson A. How to measure the QT interval-what is normal? *Am J Cardiol* 1993; 72: 14B–16B.

26 Puddu PE, Jouve R, Mariotti S, Giampaoli S, Lanti M, Reale A, Menotti A. Evaluation of 10 QT prediction formulas in 881 middle-age man from the seven countries study: emphasis on the cubic root Fridericia's equation. *J Electrocardiol* 1988; 21: 219–29.

27 Kautzner J, Hnatkova K, Camm AJ *et al*. Dependence of resting QTc interval on clinical characteristics of survivors of acute myocardial infarction: comparison of rate correction formulae. *Pacing Clin Electrophysiol* 1997; 19: 334.

28 Bazett HC. An analysis of the time-relations of electrocardiograms. *Heart: A Journal for the study of the circulation* 1920; VII: 353–70.

29 Fridericia LS. EKG systolic duration in normal subjects and heart disease patients. *Acta Med Scan* 1920; 53: 469–88.

30 Mayeda I. On time relation between systolic duration of heart and pulse rate. *Acta Scholae Med U University Imp Kioto* 1934; 17: 53.

31 Kawataki M, Kashima T, Toda H, Tanaka H. Relation between QT interval and hear rate. Applications and limitations of Bazett's formula. *J Electrocardiol* 1984; 17: 371–5.

32 Yoshinaga M, Tomari T, Aihoshi S *et al*. Exponential correction of QT interval to minimize the effect of the heart rate in children. *Jpn Circ J* 1993; 57: 102–8.

33 Boudoulas H, Geleris P, Lewis R, Rittgers SE. Linear relationship between electrical systole, mechanical systole, and heart rate. *Chest* 1981; 80: 613–7.

34 Ashman R. The normal duration of the Q-T interval. *Am Heart J* 1942: 522–34.

35 Adams W. *The normal duration of the electrocardiographic ventricular complex*. Thesis, the Department of Medicine, University of Chicago; 335–42.

36 Ljung O. A simple formula for clinical interpretation of the QT interval. *Acta Med Scand* 1949; 134: 79–86.

37 Schlamowitz I. An analysis of the relationships within the cardiac cycle in electrocardiograms of normal men. The Duration Q-T Interval its Relationship Cycle Length (R-R Interval). *Am Heart J* 1946; 31: 329–42.

38 Simonson E, Cady LD, Woodbury M. The normal Q-T interval. *Am Heart J* 1962; 63 (6): 747–53.

39 Sagie A, Larson MG, Goldberg RJ, Bengtson JR, Levy D. An improved method for adjusting the QT interval for hear rate (the Framingham Heart Study). *Am J Cardiol* 1992; 70: 797–801.

40 Akhras F, Rickards AF. The relationship between QT interval and heart rate during physiological exercise and pacing. *Jap Heart J* 1981; 22 (3): 345–51.

41 Rickards AF, Norman J. Relation between QT interval and heart rate: new design of physiologically adaptive cardiac pacemaker. *Br Heart J* 1981; 45: 56–61.

42 Hodges M, Salerno D, Erlien D. Bazett's QT correction reviewed: evidence that a linear QT correction for heart rate is better. *J Am Coll Cardiol* 1983; 1 (2): 694.

43 Kligfield P, Lax KG, Okin PM. QTc behavior during treadmill exercise as a function of the underlying QT-heart rate relationship. *J Electrocardiol* 1995; 28 (Suppl.): 206–10.

44 Wohlfart B, Pahlm O. Normal values for QT interval in ECG during ramp exercise on bicycle. *Clin Physiol* 1994; 14: 371–7.

45 Karjalainen J, Viitasalo M, manttari M, Manninen V. Relation between QT intervals and heart rates from 40 to 120 beats/min in rest electrocardiograms of men and a simple method to adjust QT interval values. *J Am Coll Cardiol* 1994; 23 (7): 1547–53.

46 Rautaharju PM, Zhou SH, Wong S, Prineas R, Berenson GS. Functional characteristics of QT prediction formulas, the concepts of QTmax and QT rate sensitivity. *Computer Biomed Res* 1993; 26: 188–204.

47 Rautaharju PM, Warren JW, Calhoum HP. Estimation of QT prolongation. A persistent, avoidable error in computer electrocardiography. *J Electrocardiol* 1990; 23 (Suppl.): 111–7.

48 Kovacs SJ Jr. The durationof the QT interval as a function of heart rate: a derivation based on physical principals and a comparison to measured values. *Am Heart J* 1985; 110: 872–8.

49 Arrowood JA, Kline J, Simpson PM, Quigg RJ, Pippin JJ, Nixon JV, Mohanty PK. Modulation of the QT interval: effects of graded exercise and reflex cardiovascular stimulation. *J Appl Physiol* 1993; 75: 2217–23.

50 Sarma JSM, Sarma RJ, Bilitch M, Katz D, Song SL. An exponential formula for heart rate dependence of QT interval during exercise and pacing in humans: reevaluation of Bazett's formula. *Am J Cardiol* 1984; 54: 103–8.

51 Lecocq B, Lecocq V, Jaillon P. Physiologic relation between cardiac cycle and QT duration in healthy volunteers. *Am J Cardiol* 1989; 63: 481–6.

52 Hodges M. Rate correction of the QT interval. *Cardiac Electrophysiol Rev* 1997; 1: 360–3.

53 Malik M. If Dr Bazett had had a computer. … *Pacing Clin Electrophysiol* 1996; 19: 1635–9.

54 Hnatkova K, Malik M. "Optimum" Formulae for Heart Rate Correction of the QT Interval. *Pacing Clin Electrophysiol* 1999; 22: 1683–7.

55 Batchvarov VN, Ghuran A, Smetana P, Hnatkova K, Harries M, Dilaveris P, Camm AJ, Malik M. QT-RR relationship in healthy subjects exhibits substantial intersubject variability and intrasubject stability. *Am J Physiol Heart Circ Physiol* 2000; 282: H2356–63.

56 European Agency for the Evaluation of Medicinal Products. Human Medicines Evaluation Unit. Committee from Proprietary Medicinal Products (CPMP). Points to consider: The assessment of the potential for QT interval prolongation by noncardiovascular medicinal products March 1997 (CPMP/986/96).

57 Nguyen PT, Scheinman MM, Seger J. Polymorphous ventricular tachycardia. clinical characterization, therapy, and the QT interval. *Circulation* 1986; 74: 340–9.

58 Makkar RR, Fromm BS, Steinman RT, Meissner MD, Lehmann MH. Female gender as a risk factor for torsades de pointes associated with cardiovascular drugs. *JAMA* 1993; 270 (21): 2590–7.

59 Bonate PL, Russell T. Assessment of QTc prolongation for noncardiac-related drugs from a drug development perspective. *J Clin Pharmacol* 1999; 39: 349–58.

60 Woosley R, Sale MQT. interval. a measure of drug action. *Am J Cardiol* 1993; 72: 36B–43B.

61 Roden DM. Torsades de Pointes. *Clin Cardiol* 1993; 16: 683–6.

62 Hii JTY, Wyse DG, Gillis AM, Duff HJ, Solylo MA, Mitchell LB. Precordial QT interval dispersion as a marker of torsades de pointes. *Circulation* 1992; 86: 1376–82.

63 Cui G, Sager PT, Singh BN, Sen L. Different effects of amiodarone and quinidine on the homogeneity of myocardial refractoriness in patients with intraventricular conduction delay. *J Cardiovasc Pharmacol Ther* 1998; 3 (3): 201–8.

64 Cui G, Sen L, Sager P, Uppal P, Singh BN. Effects of amiodarone, sematilide, and sotalol on QT dispersion. *Am J Cardiol* 1994; 74 (9): 896–900.

65 Dritsas A, Gilligan D, Nihoyannopoulos P, Oakley CM. Amiodarone reduces QT dispersion in patients with hypertrophic cardiomyopathy. *Int J Cardiol* 1992; 36: 345–9.

66 Meierhenrich R, Helguera ME, Kidwell GA, Tebbe U. Influence of amiodarone on QT dispersion in patients with life-threatening ventricular arrhythmias and clinical outcome. *Int J Cardiol* 1997; 60: 289–94.

67 Grimm W, Steder U, Menz V, Hoffmann J, Maisch B. Effect of amiodarone on QT dispersion in the 12-lead standard electrocardiogram and its significance for subsequent arrhythmic events. *Clin Cardiol* 1997; 20: 107–10.

68 Hohnloser SH, van de Loo A, Baedeker F. Efficacy and proarrhythmic hazards of pharmacologic cardioversion of atrial fibrillation: prospective comparison of sotalol versus quinidine. *J Am Coll Cardiol* 1995; 26: 852–8.

69 Houltz B, Darpo B, Edvardsson N *et al.* Electrocardiographic and clinical predictors of torsades de pointes induced by almokalant infusion in patients with chronic atrial fibrillation or flutter: a prospective study. *Pacing Clin Electrophysiol* 1998; 21 (5): 1044–57.

70 Day CP, McComb JM, Mathews J, Campbell RWF. Reduction in QT dispersion by sotalol following myocardial infarction. *Eur Heart J* 1991; 12: 423–7.

71 Hohnloser SH, van de loo A, kalusche D *et al.* Does sotalol-induced alteration of QT dispersion predict drug effectiveness or pro-arrhythmic hazards? *Circulation* 1993; 88 (Suppl. I): 397 (Abstract).

72 Murray A, McLaughlin NB, Campbell RW. Measuring QT dispersion: man versus machine. *Heart* 1997; 77: 539–42.

73 Malik M, Batchvarov V. QT dispersion in normal subjects and in the general population 2000 *Malik M and Batchvarov V, QT Dispersion. Futura*, New York, pp. 55–63.

74 Perkiomaki JS, Koistinen MJ, Yli-Mayry S, Huikuri HV. Dispersion of QT interval in patients with and without susceptibility to ventricular tachyarrhythmias after previous myocardial infarction. *J Am Coll Cardiol* 1995; 26: 174–9.

75 Glancy JM, Garratt CJ, Woods KL, de Bono DP. QT dispersion and mortality after myocardial infarction. *Lancet* 1995; 345: 945–8.

76 Zabel M, Klingenheben T, Franz MR, Hohnloser SH. Assessment of QT dispersion for prediction of mortality or arrhythmic events after myocardial infarction. Results of a prospective, long-term follow-up study. *Circulation* 1998; 97: 2543–50.

77 Malik M, Batchvarov V. Effect of drugs on QT dispersion and the risk of torsades de pointes tachycardia 2000 In: Malik M, Batchvarov V, eds. *QT Dispersion.* Futura, New York, pp. 46–54.

78 Barr CS, Naas A, Freeman M, Lang CC, Struthers AD. QT dispersion and sudden unexpected death in chronic heart failure. *Lancet* 1994; 343: 327–9.

79 Day CP, McComb JM, Campbell RWF. QT dispersion: an indication of arrhythmic risk in patients with long QT intervals. *Br Heart J* 1990; 63: 342–4.

80 Acar B, Yi G, Hnatkova K, Malik M. Spatial, temporal and wavefront direction characteristics of 12-lead T wave morphology. *Med Biol Eng Comput* 1999; 37: 1–11.

81 Morganroth J, Brozovich FV, McDonald JT, Jacobs RA. Variability of the QT measurement in healthy men, with implications for selection of an abnormal QT value to predict drug toxicity and proarrhythmia. *Am J Cardiol* 1991; 67: 774–6.

82 Gunput MD, Williams P, Yogendran L, Keene ON, Maconochie JG. QTc, PR interval and heart rate variability in healthy volunteer-a review of 12-lead ECG data from clinical pharmacology studies. *Br J Clin Pharmacol* 1995; 39: 577P.

83 Sharma PP, Sarma JSM, Singh BN. Effects of sotalol on the circadian rhythmicity of heart rate and QT intervals with a noninvasive index of reverse-use dependency. *J Cardiovasc Pharmacol Therapeut* 1999; 4 (1): 15–21.

84 Bexton RS, Vallin HO, Camm AJ. Diurnal variation of the QT interval. *Br Heart J* 1986; 55: 253–8.

85 Pratt CM, Ruberg S, Morganroth J *et al.* Dose–response relation between terfenadine (Seldene) and the Qtc interval on the scalar electrocardiogram: distinguishing drug effect from spontaneous variability. *Am Heart J* 1996; 131: 472–80.

86 Alexopoulos D, Rynkiewicz A, Yusuf S, Johnston JA, Sleight P, Yacoub MH. Diurnal variations of QT interval after cardiac transplantation. *Am J Cardiol* 1988; 62: 482–5.

87 Buckingham TA, Bhutto ZR, Telfer EA, Zbilut J. Differences in corrected QT intervals at minimal and maximal heart rate may identify patients at risk for torsades de pointes during treatment with antiarrhythmic drugs. *J Cardiovasc Electrophysiol* 1994; 5 (5): 408–11.

88 Kadish AH, Weisman HF, Veltri EP, Epstein AE, Slepian MJ, Levine JH. Paradoxical effects of exercise on the QT interval in patients with polymorphic ventricular tachycardia receiving type Ia antiarrhythmic agents. *Circulation* 1990; 81 (1): 14–9.

89 Antimisiaris M, Sarma JSM, Schoenbaum MP, Sharma PP, Venkataraman K, Singh BN, Christenson P. Effects of amiodarone on the circadian rhythm and power spectral changes of heart rate and QT interval: significance for the control of sudden cardiac death. *Am Heart J* 1994; 128: 884–91.

CHAPTER 4

Introduction to drug-induced long QT syndrome

Drug effects are the most common cause of acquired long QT syndrome (LQTS). Many drugs are known to prolong the QT interval, with antiarrhythmics being most commonly implicated. In recent years, it has become apparent that a spectrum of noncardiac drugs such as nonsedating antihistamines, macrolide antibiotics, antipsychotics, and others can cause QT prolongation and aggravate TdP [1]. Of concern is that the proarrhythmic risk of many of these drugs was not detected during the developmental phase and was recognized only after the drug had been marketed for many years.

Incidence of drug-induced torsades de pointes

The number of drugs associated with QT prolongation and TdP is increasing and may continue to do so, particularly with the development of highly targeted pure class III antiarrhythmic drugs. This issue has been identified as a considerable public health problem and has attracted attention and concern from the drug regulatory authorities leading to drug withdrawals. The view that drug-induced QT prolongation and TdP is usually an intrinsic effect of a whole therapeutic class (e.g., class III antiarrhythmics) is often unjustified as in many cases, it is displayed only by some compounds within a given class of nonantiarrhythmic drugs (e.g., nonsedating antihistamines). Drug-induced QT prolongation and/or TdP are sometimes considered idiosyncratic, totally unpredictable adverse drug reactions, but a number of risk factors for their occurrence are well recognized. In addition, many published case reports or case series on drug-induced proarrhythmias are inadequate, and some of them only involve extreme overdosage and cannot be directly extrapolated to routine clinical practice. In others, the coadministration of medications that may also prolong the QT interval renders it impossible to establish a causal relationship between a single drug and the occurrence of QT prolongation and/or TdP. Finally, while it has been recognized that virtually all QT-prolonging drugs share the potential to block the myocardial voltage-gated rapid component of the delayed rectifier potassium current (I_{Kr}), which is the basic mechanism for their proarrhythmic effects (see Chapter 2), they do not necessarily cause noticeable QT prolongation in all individuals. At times, when the electrocardiographic signs are not evident, the underlying blockade of I_{Kr} current may be sufficient to precipitate the occurrence of arrhythmia. Thus, the identification of offending drugs that may present a serious proarrhythmic risk remains an enormous clinical and scientific challenge.

In a survey in both the UK and Italy, noncardiac drugs that have proarrhythmic potential (i.e., official warning on QT prolongation or TdP, or with published data on QT prolongation, ventricular tachycardia or class III effect) represented 3% and 2% of total prescriptions in both countries, respectively [2]. The danger of drug-induced proarrhythmia is therefore serious. It is prudent that all physicians who prescribe these drugs, and patients who receive them, should be aware of this risk and take the precautions to minimize proarrhythmia. Widespread knowledge of the risk factors and the implementation of a comprehensive listing of QT-prolonging drugs have become important issues.

The exact incidence of drug-induced TdP in the general population is largely unknown. Most of our understanding of the incidence, risk factors and drug interaction of proarrhythmic drugs is derived from epidemiological studies, anecdotal case reports, clinical studies during drug development and postmarketing surveillance. The awareness of drug-induced TdP in the last few years has resulted in an increase in the number of spontaneous reports. Nevertheless, the absolute total number remains very low although it has been suggested that the system of spontaneous reporting under-reports the true incidence of serious adverse reactions by a factor of at least 10 [3]. Between 1983 and December 1999, 761 cases of TdP, of which 34 were fatal, were reported to the WHO Drug Monitoring Center by the member states. The WHO data provide an insight into the incidence of TdP with the most commonly reported proarrhythmic drugs [4] [Table 4.1]. However, such a reporting system is undermined by the widely variable content and clinical information between different countries and sources. It is also compounded by various factors such as the patient's underlying disease, whether the adverse drug reaction is well known or not previously described and the amount of attention paid by the medical community to a specific adverse drug reaction. For instance, the cases of TdP that had been associated with digoxin use could have been due to bradycardia, either as a result of digoxin or an underlying bradyarrhythmia, as digoxin is not known to block the I_{Kr} channel and thereby cause QT prolongation. The WHO database does not provide information relevant to co-factors and other etiologies for TdP.

Classification of torsadogenic potency of drugs

The quantification and comparison of the risk of TdP among the proarrhythmic drugs are difficult. The torsadogenic potency of drugs is extremely variable, even within the same class of drugs. For instance, some drugs may only provoke TdP in the setting of overdose, concomitant administration of other QT-prolonging drugs, or in the presence of risk factors such as hypokalemia; whereas others may induce TdP alone, even at therapeutic

Table 4.1 Twenty most commonly reported drugs associated with TdP between 1983 and 1999 (reproduced from [4]).

Drug	TdP (n)	Fatal (n)	Total (n)	TdP/total (%)
Sotalol	130	1	2758	4.71
Cisapride	97	6	6489	1.49
Amiodarone	47	1	13725	0.34
Erythromycin	44	2	24776	0.18
Ibutilide	43	1	173	24.86
Terfenadine	41	1	10047	0.41
Quinidine	33	2	7353	0.45
Clarithromycin	33	0	17448	0.19
Haloperidol	21	6	15431	0.14
Fluoxetine	20	1	70929	0.03
Digoxin	19	0	18925	0.10
Procainamide	19	0	5867	0.32
Terodiline	19	0	2248	0.85
Fluconazole	17	0	5613	0.30
Disopyramide	16	1	3378	0.47
Bepridil	15	0	384	3.91
Furosemide	15	0	15119	0.10
Thioridazine	12	0	6565	0.18
Flecainide	11	2	3747	0.29
Loratidine	11	1	5452	0.20

TdP (n), total number of adverse drug reactions reports named TdP for this drug; Fatal (n), number of adverse drug reactions reports named TdP with fatal outcome; Total (n), total number of adverse drug reactions reports for drug.

(or subtherapeutic) level, and in the absence of coexisting risk factors. Thus, a system is needed whereby a distinction can be made when reporting on the torsadogenic risk of the particular drug(s), taking into account all available evidence. The current system of reporting and assessing the proarrhythmic potential of a QT-prolonging drug is less than perfect. For instance, although the published clinical trials represent a major source of clinical evidence, it is limited by publication bias, especially "negative" studies are hard to publish [5]. Molecular studies on cardiac repolarization are helpful in studying the arrhythmogenic mechanism of a drug suspected of prolonging ventricular repolarization, but it is difficult to extrapolate the *in vitro* studies into clinical relevance. No model has an absolute predictive value [5]. The official warnings from drug regulatory authorities, such as the United States Food and Drug Administration or the United Kingdom Medicines and Healthcare Products Regulatory Agency, provide easily available sources of information for physicians, often on data that are not available as published data, but they are not always updated and frequently reflect precautions taken at the time of marketing authorization. For example, they may consider QT prolongation as a class effect rather than an effect displayed only by some compounds within the class of drugs.

In an attempt to provide a systematic classification of QT-prolonging drugs, Haverkamp *et al.* proposed a classification of the torsadogenic potency of proarrhythmic drugs [6]. The classification is summarized in Table 4.2. The major criterion for classification is the potency of a drug to provoke TdP.

Table 4.2 Classification of torsadogenic potency of drugs (adapted from [6]).

Classification	Features
Class A (High torsadogenic potency)	• Potent blockers of repolarization currents • Documented prolongation of APD & induction of EAD • Documented QT prolongation and cases of TdP at therapeutic doses/concentration by the drug alone in the absence of coadministration of QT-prolonging drugs or risk factors • The IC_{50} for the prolongation of repolarization is in the same range as the IC_{50} for the therapeutic action
Class B (Medium torsadogenic potency)	• Drugs that prolong myocardial repolarization (i.e., APD and QT interval) at higher doses, or at normal doses with coadministration of drugs that inhibit drug metabolism (e.g., by inhibiting the cytochrome P450 system) • The IC_{50} for the prolongation of repolarization is above the IC_{50} for the therapeutic action • Cases of TdP induced by the drug alone have been documented but TdP is usually associated with metabolic inhibition and/or the presence of other risk factors
Class C (Low torsadogenic potency)	• Drugs that prolong APD and QT interval at high doses/concentration clearly above therapeutic range • The effect of repolarization manifests only during overdose, intoxication or in the presence of severe metabolic inhibition • Cases of TdP have been documented but in the presence of risk factors
Class D (Torsadogenic potential unclear)	• Drugs that block repolarizing ion currents *in vitro* but which have so far not been shown to prolong repolarization in other *in vitro* models (e.g., papillary muscle fibers or isolated hearts) or the concentrations necessary for this effect were far above the clinical concentrations • Prolongation of the human QT interval has not been demonstrated in systematic randomized studies • Cases of the TdP in association with treatment with the drug may have been reported but the causal relation between the event and the drug is not clear

It is important to understand that this system does not assume that all drugs under the same class exert the identical risk ratio in their torsadogenic potency, as clearly it will never be possible to a have a head-to-head comparison of the proarrhythmic potency of, for example, antiarrhythmic drugs vs. quinolone antibiotics. This is merely an attempt to give a measure of proportion and comparison in the risks among various proarrhythmic drugs. Furthermore, this classification has a drawback in that published data on the effect on the QT intervals, I_{Kr} channel and propensity to induce early after-depolarizations are not available for all drugs that may cause TdP. Thus, this classification should be a dynamic system and the assignment of a drug to a particular torsadogenic class may change over time depending on the available knowledge. We have listed the drugs that have been documented to be torsadogenic in the literature in Table 4.3 and classified the risk using the system proposed by Haverkamp *et al.*

Table 4.3 Drugs that can prolong QT interval and/or induce TdP.

Class of drugs	Drugs	Torsadogenic risk
Antiarrhythmic drugs	Type 1A (TdP reported in all)	
	Ajmaline (TdP reported)	A
	Disopyramide (TdP reported)	A
	Procainamide (TdP reported)	A
	Quinidine (TdP reported)	A
	Type 1C (increase QT by prolonging QRS interval)	
	Encainide	D
	Flecainide	D
	Moracizine	D
	Propafenone	D
	Type 3 (TdP reported in all)	
	Amiodarone	B
	Dronedarone	D
	d'l-Sotalol	A
	d-Sotalol	A
	Bretylium	A
	Azimilide	A
	Dofetilide	A
	Ersentilide	D
	Ibutilide	A
	Trecetilide	D
	Tedisamil	A
	Almokalant	A
Calcium channel blocker	Prenylamine (TdP reported, withdrawn)	A
	Bepridil (TdP reported, withdrawn)	A
	Mibefradil	A
	Terodiline (TdP reported, withdrawn)	A

(Continued)

Table 4.3 (*Continued*)

Class of drugs	Drugs	Torsadogenic risk
Psychiatric drugs	Chlorpromazine (TdP reported)	C
	Thioridazine (TdP reported)	A
	Droperidol (TdP reported)	A
	Haloperidol (TdP reported)	A
	Amitriptyline	B
	Nortriptyline	B
	Clomipramine	B
	Desipramine (TdP reported)	B
	Imipramine (TdP reported)	B
	Maprotiline (TdP reported)	A
	Chloral hydrate	C
	Doxepin (TdP reported)	B
	Lithium (TdP reported)	D
	Pimozide (TdP reported)	A
	Sertindole (TdP reported)	A
	Ziprasidone	C/D
Antihistamines	Astemizole (TdP reported)	A
	Terfenadine (TdP reported)	A
	Diphenhydramine	D
	Ebastine	C/D
	Mizolastine	C
Antimicrobial and antimalarial drugs	Clarithromycin (TdP reported)	A
	Erythromycin, intravenous (TdP reported)	A
	Roxithromycin (TdP reported)	B
	Josamycin	D
	Erythromycylamine	D
	Oleandomycin	D
	Fluconazole (TdP reported)	B
	Itraconazole (TdP reported when used with other QT prolonging drugs)	B
	Ketoconazole	B
	Miconazoles	B
	Grepafloxacin (TdP reported, withdrawn worldwide)	A
	Sparfloxacin (TdP reported)	A
	Levofloxacin (TdP reported)	B
	Moxifloxacin (TdP reported)	D
	Gatifloxacin (TdP reported)	D
	Ciprofloxacin (TdP reported)	D
	Chloroquine (TdP reported)	D
	Halofantrine (TdP reported)	A
	Quinine (TdP reported)	A
	Pentamidine (TdP reported)	A
	Pentavalent antimonial meglumine (TdP reported)	A
Prokinetics (serotonin agonists)	Cisapride (TdP reported, withdrawn in the US & UK	A

(*Continued p. 66*)

Table 4.3 (*Continued*)

Class of drugs	Drugs	Torsadogenic risk
5HT$_2$ serotonin antagonist	Ketanserin (TdP reported, withdrawn in the US & UK)	A
Dopamine-receptor antagonist	Domperidone (intravenous)	A
Immunosuppressant	Tacrolimus (TdP reported)	A
Antidiuretic hormone	Vasopressin (TdP reported)	B
Other agents	Adenosine (TdP reported)	D
	Organophosphates (TdP reported)	C
	Papaverine (intracoronary) (TdP reported)	A
	Probucol (TdP reported)	B
	Cocaine	C
	Arsenic trioxide (TdP reported)	A

Disclaimer: this list is not comprehensive and the classification of the torsadogenic risk with individual drugs is proposed by the authors is based on information available in the literature at the time of preparation of this book. The authors disclaim any liability, loss, injury, or damage incurred as a consequence, directly or indirectly, of the use and application of any of the contents of this table. The information presented on this table is intended as general health information and as an educational tool. It is not intended as medical advice, nor is it necessarily consistent with regulatory statements and drug labelling.

Redfern and colleagues also attempted to assess the proarrhythmic risk of drugs [7]. They first categorized the drugs according to their torsadogenic propensity, then collected and tabulated the information on effective free plasma therapeutic concentration (ETPCunbound) with inhibition of HERG/IKr current, effects on cardiac action potential duration *in vitro*, prolongation of QT interval in dogs, and QT prolongation in man. It is hoped that by presenting all these data together, their classification system will provide some clarification on pre-clinical detection on torsadogenic propensity and evidence for setting a provisional safety margin. The classification system was summarized in Fig. 4.1. In addition, this study also confirmed that most drugs that are associated with TdP in humans are associated with the blockade of HERG channel at a concentration close to or superimposed upon the free plasma concentration found in clinical use. Interactions with multiple cardiac ion channels can either mitigate or exacerbate the prolongation of action potential duration and QT interval that would ensue from the blockade of IKr current alone, and delay of repolarization per se is not necessarily torsadogenic. Finally, an integrated assessment of *in vitro* and *in vivo* data is required in order to predict the torsadogenic risk of a new drug in humans.

In the following few chapters, we will provide an overview of the different classes of drugs reported to prolong the QT interval and/or induce TdP, give some insight on the proarrhythmic risks among drugs of the same class and discuss the clinical relevance of their proarrhythmic cardiotoxicity.

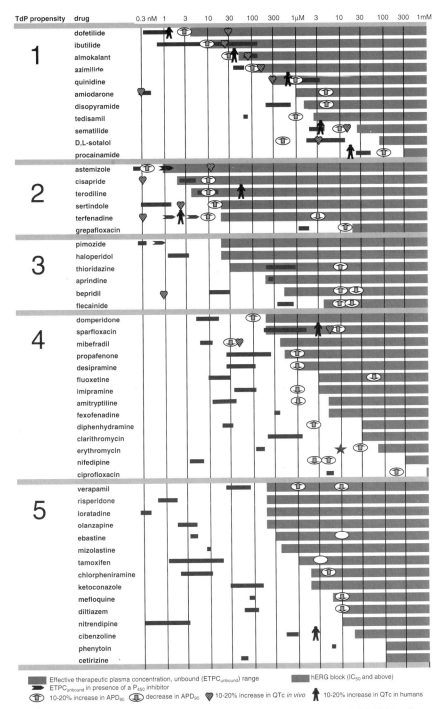

Fig. 4.1 Relationships between clinical plasma concentrations (unbound), hERG inhibition (from IC50 upwards), prolongation of APD90, QT prolongation *in vivo* and QT prolongation in man for 52 drugs across all 5 Categories. (Courtesy of Dr WS Redfern, reproduced with permission.)

References

1 Malik M, Camm AJ. Evaluation of drug-induced QT interval prolongation: implications for drug approval and labelling. *Drug Safety* 2001; 24: 324–51.

2 De Ponti F, Poluzzi E, Montanaro N, Ferguson. J. QTc and psychotropic drugs. *Lancet* 2000; 356 (9223): 75–6.

3 Wysowski DK, Bacsanyi. J. Cisapride and fatal arrhythmia. *N Engl J Med* 1996; 335: 290–1.

4 Darpo B. Spectrum of drugs prolonging QT interval and the incidence of torsades de pointes. *Eur Heart J* 2001; 3 (Suppl. K): K70–K80.

5 De Ponti F, Poluzzi E. Organizing evidence on QT prolongation and occurrence of Torsades de Pointes with nonantiarrhythmic drugs: a call for consensus. *Eur J Clin Pharmacol* 2001; 57: 185–209.

6 Haverkamp W, Eckardt L, Monnig G, Schulze-Bahr E, Wadekind H, Kirchhof P, Haverkamp F, Breithardt G. Clinical aspects of ventricular arrhythmias associated with QT prolongation. *Eur Heart J* 2001; 3 (Suppl. K): K81–K88.

7 Redfern WS, Carlsson L, Davis AS *et al*. Relationships between preclinical cardiac electrophysiology, clinical QT interval prolongation and torsade de pointes for a broad range of drugs: evidence for a provisional safety margin in drug development. *Cardiovasc Res* 2003; 58(1): 32–45.

CHAPTER 5

Risk of QT prolongation and torsades de pointes with antiarrhythmic drugs

Introduction

The concept that certain arrhythmias, especially atrial and ventricular fibrillation, might be controlled by prolonging myocardial refractoriness has long been recognized and much interest has been concentrated on the development of antiarrhythmic drugs (AADs) with this action [1]. However, it is now recognized that antiarrhythmic drugs that prolong ventricular repolarization may provoke or aggravate the occurrence of TdP. If rapid or prolonged, this can lead to ventricular fibrillation and sudden cardiac death. Antiarrhythmic agents are probably the best-studied and most common causes of drug-induced acquired long QT syndrome and TdP.

The arrhythmogenic mechanism of AADs is still not well understood. In quinidine-induced TdP, arrhythmia formation may be dependent on bradycardia, hypokalaemia and prolongation of the QT interval. This suggests that AAD-induced TdP is principally a disorder of repolarization. There were several initial suggested mechanisms for the arrhythmia [2] which included:

1 ventricular activation caused by a minimum of two automatic foci interacting at slightly different rate;

2 localized re-entry resulting from an increased disparity of action potential duration (refractoriness) following drug administration, with the U wave representing delayed repolarization in Purkinje fibers; and

3 bradycardia-dependent triggering of ventricular arrhythmia from after-depolarizations, with the U wave representing the temporal summation of early after-depolarizations.

It is now recognized that blockade of the normal outward rapid component of the delayed rectifier potassium current, I_{Kr}, or abnormal prolongation of inward current carried by sodium or calcium channels, or the simultaneous operation of enhanced inward and reduced outward currents by AADs results in the prolongation of action potential duration and slowing of repolarization (see Chapter 2). The prolongation of repolarization that precedes a subsequent activation of the inward depolarization current allows re-entry and induces an abnormality in the terminal repolarization, referred to as an early after-depolarization, which is responsible for the increased amplitude of the U wave on the ECG and may promote repetitive triggered activity. When accompanied by the presence of markedly increased dispersion of repolarization, often induced by the same drug, this results in re-entry and provoke TdP, which is then sustained by further re-entry or spiral wave activity. Such phenomena are more readily induced in the His–Purkinje network and mid-myocardial (M) cells.

Despite the discovery that the blockade of I_{Kr} potassium channels is often essential for drug-induced QT prolongation and TdP, the mechanisms underlying AAD-induced proarrhythmia is far from understood. As TdP occurs in the setting of a long QT interval, its basis is given as a possible sequel of antiarrhythmic drugs that prolong ventricular refractoriness. However, the proarrhythmic potential varies between AADs that prolong the QT interval. It is well known that the incidence of TdP resulting from quinidine has a poor correlation with the serum drug level. In contrast, there is a direct correlation between sotalol dosage and the incidence of TdP. Amiodarone, on the other hand, has a very low incidence of TdP despite its marked effects on the QT interval. The discordance between QT prolongation and the incidence of TdP among antiarrhythmic drugs that prolong ventricular refractoriness has presented a challenge in the understanding of proarrhythmic vs. antiarrhythmic drug mechanism, particularly with regard to the design of future antiarrhythmic drug.

In the last decade, the development of class III drugs has been the core interest in the search for an ideal antiarrhythmic drug, especially after the publication of studies documenting that certain class I drugs may increase mortality in high-risk postinfarction patients. Class III drugs lack negative hemodynamic effects, can affect both atrial and ventricular tissue, and can be administered as either parenteral or oral preparations [1]. However, the development of the so-called "pure class III drugs" that only prolong the cardiac repolarization and refractoriness without other pharmacologic effect has met with some disappointment, not least because of their proarrhythmic effect.

Class I antiarrhythmics

Quinidine

Although the Vaughan-Williams classification of antiarrhythmic drugs may seem to imply that only class III drugs block I_{Kr} channels and prolong the action potential duration, many class Ia drugs also show I_{Kr}-channel-blocking property. Quinidine affects depolarization and repolarization by blocking both sodium and potassium channels. It blocks the delayed rectifier I_{Kr} [3], as well as I_{Ks} channels, although the relevance of I_{Ks} blockade in the risk of TdP is unclear. Experimentally, quinidine induces early after-depolarizations with prolongation of the action potential, during bradycardia and hypokalemia. The early landmark report by Selzer and Wray observed that quinidine use was associated with syncope (so-called "quinidine syncope") and ventricular fibrillation/flutter but it was not until many years after its introduction that an association between quinidine and TdP was described [4]. TdP with class Ia drugs can occur at therapeutic, low therapeutic or subtherapeutic concentrations [4,5]. It has been suggested that perhaps the blockade of the sodium channel by class Ia drugs suppresses the QT prolonging effect at higher concentrations. In contrast, pure I_{Kr} potassium blockers such as d-sotalol prolong the QT interval and induce TdP at an incidence directly proportional to their concentration until the potassium currents are completely blocked [6].

Quinidine prolongs the QT by an average of 10–15%, most often early during therapy, usually within 1 week of initiation of therapy [6–8], with an incidence of TdP estimated to be at least 1.5%/year but this depends in part on the patient population treated [6]. The QT prolonging effect varies greatly among individuals and patients that develop TdP generally show much more marked changes [6]. The risk of TdP is estimated to occur in between 1 and 8.8% of patients [7,9], but can rise to 28% when prescribed to patients for the treatment of ventricular arrhythmias [10]. TdP with quinidine (or disopyramide) was described when the QTc interval was longer than 520 ms [11]. However, TdP can develop without marked prolongation of the QT interval and the plasma level of quinidine does not predict proarrhythmia. In line with other drug-induced TdP, hypokalaemia and bradycardia including heart block facilitates the development of TdP with quinidine [7,11], and this may be due to exacerbation of early afterdepolarizations with hypokalaemia and longer cycle length [12]. Interestingly, patients with TdP or syncope due to quinidine usually have heart disease [8,13] and are prescribed quinidine for the treatment of atrial fibrillation [8]. In such patients, TdP occurs predominantly in the first few hours after conversion to sinus rhythm but not during atrial fibrillation [7,14] and this may be related to the slowing in heart rate after conversion to sinus rhythm. Another explanation could be the abrupt lengthening in cycle length after atrial fibrillation is converted to sinus rhythm inducing an increase in the transmural dispersion of repolarization, which favors re-entry and TdP. Generally, TdP with class Ia drugs tends not to be dose-dependent, with the exception of procainamide.

Procainamide

Procainamide predominantly blocks the inactivated state of the sodium channel. It is metabolized in the liver to N-acetyl-procainamide (NAPA), which is active and similar to the parent drug, procainamide. NAPA exhibits class III antiarrhythmic activity by prolonging the QT interval. The change in the QT interval with procainamide does not reliably predict the occurrence of TdP [15]. However, the risk of TdP is dose-dependent, especially in patients with renal failure because both procainamide and NAPA accumulate during renal failure [16,17].

At frequently used plasma levels, procainamide prolongs the QT interval to a lesser degree than quinidine and this effect does not appear to be due to comparison of "nonequivalent" drug levels [18]. However, similarly to quinidine, procainamide can cause TdP at low therapeutic or subtherapeutic concentrations [5]. NAPA increases the QT interval by about 8% [19].

Disopyramide

Disopyramide depresses conduction by blocking the sodium channel and prolongs repolarization moderately by blocking the I_{Kr} (as well as I_{K1}, I_{Ca} and I_{to}) channels and thus induces early after-depolarizations [20]. Therefore, it can prolong the QT interval and cause TdP and ventricular fibrillation [21–23], particularly in patients with severe repolarization delay, sinus brady-cardia or atrioventricular block [21], although its propensity appears to be less than that of quinidine [24]. Disopyramide prolongs the QT interval at approximately 0.5–4 h after a single dose of 200 mg of the medication [25].

In patients with ventricular fibrillation secondary to class Ia antiarrhythmics such as disopyramide, quinidine and procainamide, the baseline QT interval was significantly longer compared to those patients without ventricular fibrillation (QTc = 470 ms vs. 440 ms), despite both groups having similar degrees of QT prolongation during drug therapy. In these patients, ventricular fibrillation is an early event, and there may be an increased risk of its recurrence with subsequent trials of antiarrhythmic drugs. Left ventricular dysfunction and concomitant therapy with digitalis or diuretic agents may predispose patients to this complication [26].

In patients with congestive heart failure, renal insufficiency and/or hepatic dysfunction, the use of disopyramide is contraindicated due to its progressive lengthening of ventricular depolarization and repolarization which has resulted in cardiovascular collapse and death in some patients [27,28].

Ajmaline

The use of ajmaline has been related to QT prolongation, QRS prolongation, A-V block, hypovolemic shock, ventricular tachycardia, TdP and cardiac arrest [29–32]. The first cardiac disturbance can appear 1 h after ingestion [30]. Ajmaline prolongs the QT interval by 17% [32]. Ajmaline suppresses the I_{Ca} current in a dose-dependent manner as well as inhibiting the inward rectifying I_{K1} current and the delayed rectifier I_{Kr} current without altering the activation or deactivation time courses. All these inhibitory effects of ajmaline prolong the action potential duration in a dose-dependent manner [33].

Class III antiarrhythmics

The majority of the class III antiarrhythmic drugs have a reverse use-dependency effect on the action potential duration, prolonging the effective refractory period of cardiac tissue more at slower heart rates. This property results from the preferential block of the rapid component of the delayed rectifier potassium current I_{Kr}, which is more active at slow heart rates. Block of this current is the major factor responsible for the increased risk of TdP associated with most class III antiarrhythmics [34].

Amiodarone

Amiodarone increases the QT interval progressively and at a constant dose reaches a steady-state effect at 6–12 months [35]. Despite the same potent effects on QT prolongation, the incidence of TdP is very low with amiodarone compared to other class III agents [36]. TdP rarely occurs during monotherapy with amiodarone over a prolonged period of time, despite QT prolongation to > 600 ms and an accompanying bradycardia of < 50 bpm. When TdP occurs with amiodarone, it usually, although not invariably, occurs during concomitant therapy with other QT prolonging drugs or in the context of severe electrolyte disturbances such as hypokalemia or bradycardia (Figs 5.1, 5.2 and 5.3).

A literature review revealed that the incidence of TdP with amiodarone was very low at only 0.7% in 17 uncontrolled studies (2878 patients) between 1982 and 1993, and no proarrhythmia was reported in seven controlled studies (1464

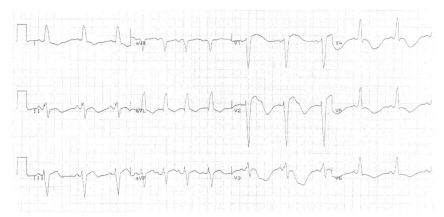

Fig. 5.1 QT prolongation on an ECG in a patient receiving amiodarone for ventricular tachyarrhythmia. Note the QTc was 692 ms with bizarre large inverted T waves. Ventricular depolarization is also abnormal.

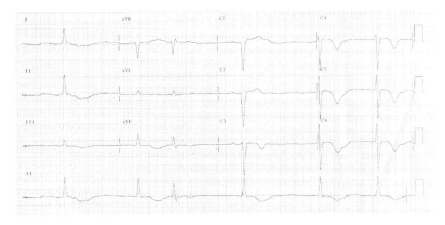

Fig. 5.2 A hypokalemic bradycardic female patient receiving amiodarone for paroxysmal atrial fibrillation developed QT prolongation and TdP. Note the large T/U wave complex.

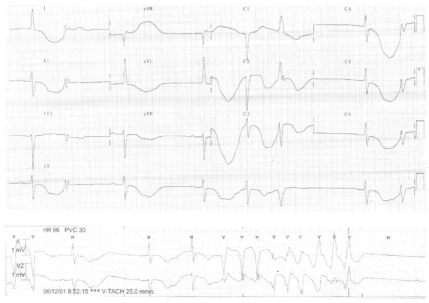

Fig. 5.3 The ECGs of an elderly female patient who developed bradycardia, severe QT prolongation (QTc interval = 590 ms) and nonsustained TdP after taking amiodarone (200 mg) for paroxysmal atrial fibrillation. The amiodarone was withdrawn and she was treated with a permanent pacemaker implantation.

patients) between 1987 and 1992 [36]. In this review, none of the patients with previous drug-induced TdP developed recurrent TdP when exposed to amiodarone despite amiodarone-induced QT prolongation equivalent to that observed at the time of TdP during exposure to previous drugs [36]. Intravenous amiodarone is also safe and effective for the treatment of ventricular tachyarrhythmias [37]. Indeed, the evidence from a recent meta-analysis of amiodarone primary prevention trials comprising 6553 patients showed that amiodarone actually reduced the risk of arrhythmic death and resuscitated cardiac arrest compared to placebo in patients after myocardial infarction or with heart failure [38]. No proarrhythmia was reported in this meta-analysis [38].

The precise mechanism for the low incidence of proarrhythmia with amiodarone is unknown. There are a number of features about the drug effect on repolarization that differ from those of class III antiarrhythmic drugs, which may account for the different proarrhythmic potential between amiodarone and other class III agents (Table 5.1) [35]. Unlike other class III antiarrhythmic drugs, amiodarone is a complex molecule in that it uniquely possesses pharmacological properties from all 4 antiarrhythmic classes. Amiodarone noncompetitively blocks sympathetic stimulation, and its effects on repolarization are not associated with reverse use dependency, despite its I_{Kr} channel blocking effect [39,40]. In addition, amiodarone also blocks the fast sodium current and the slow inward calcium current mediated through the L-calcium channels [35].

Table 5.1 Possible mechanisms accounting for the different proarrhythmic potentials of amiodarone, sotalol, and pure class III antiarrhythmic drugs (AAD) in causing TdP (modified from [35]).

Effect	Amiodarone	Sotalol	Pure class III AAD
Bradycadia	↑↑	↑↑↑	+/−
QT/QTc prolongation	↑↑↑	↑↑	↑↑
repolarization dispersion			
Spatial	↓↓	↓→+/−	+/−?↑
Temporal	↓↓	?	?
EAD generation in PF or M cells	↓↓	↑	↑↑
Reverse use/rate dependency of APD	−	↑	↑↑
Calcium channel antagonism	++	−	−
K⁺ dependency of APD	+/−	↑↑	↑↑
T3 interaction	++	−	−
Incidence of TdP	<1%	3–4%	3–6%

⊥, variable effects; ↑, increase; ↓, decrease; −, absent; +, present; AAD, antiarrhythmic drug; APD, action potential duration; EAD, early after-depolarization; K⁺, potassium; PF, Purkinje fibers; T3, triiodothyronine.

The calcium channel-blocking action of amiodarone is thought to prevent the development of calcium-dependent early after-depolarizations and triggered activity, hence minimizing the risk of TdP [35]. Furthermore, amiodarone reduces the temporal and spatial dispersion of repolarization, and might improve the homogeneity of refractoriness, thereby reducing the possibility of focal excitation and TdP [38]. Finally, amiodarone is also a coronary vasodilator, an anti-ischemic drug and an antifibrillatory agent.

d,l-Sotalol

Racemic sotalol is a beta-adrenergic blocking agent that prolongs the duration of the cardiac action potential without affecting the upstroke velocity of depolarization. d,l-Sotalol is a racemic drug composed of equimolar amounts of its stereoisomers, d-(+)-sotalol and l-(−)-sotalol. The l-(−) enantiomer has both beta-blocking (class II) activity and potassium-channel-blocking (class III) properties. The d-(+) enantiomer has class III properties but only 1/50 of the beta-blocking activity of the l-(−) enantiomer. Both d,l-sotalol and d-sotalol block the delayed rectifier I_{Kr} potassium current (hence, the risk of QT prolongation and TdP), with no effect on the slow component I_{Ks} current [41]. They have minimal effect on the inward rectifier current [41]. d,l-Sotalol has the additional beta-blocking effect, resulting in an important bradycardic effect.

d,l-Sotalol prolongs the QT interval in a dose- and concentration-dependent manner and decreases at rapid heart rates. At a given plasma concentration, QT interval prolongation during repeated dosing tends to be less pronounced than QT prolongation at the same plasma concentration during single dosing [42]. Proarrhythmia with d,l-sotalol occurs primarily within the first 3 days of dosing [43], and the incidence of TdP increases with the dose and baseline values of the QT interval [44]. The incidence rate of TdP with a daily dose of 80–160 mg of d,l-sotalol was estimated to be approximately 0.5%, which rises to 6.8% for a daily dose of >640 mg [44]. However, the risk of TdP is also dependent on the risk of the population treated and is greater in patients with congestive heart failure and low ejection fraction. The overall risk of TdP has been estimated to be around 0.5% in all patients treated (including patients given d,l-sotalol for atrial fibrillation, supraventricular tachycardia, angina, hypertension or other conditions) [45]. In patients treated for the control of sustained ventricular tachyarrhythmias, the risk of TdP is high and is estimated to be between 4.1 and 5%. TdP have occurred early during treatment even with low doses of oral d,l-sotalol [45,46]. Renal failure leads to accumulation of d, l-sotalol and increases the risk of TdP.

Pure class III antiarrhythmic agents

d-Sotalol

In contrast to the racemic compound, d-sotalol is devoid of clinically relevant antiadrenergic activity. It can be considered as the prototype pure class III antiarrhythmic agent because of its major blocking effect on the I_{Kr} channel. As a result, like the rest of the pure class III antiarrhythmics, d-sotalol prolongs the action potential and the corresponding effective refractory period without influencing the pacing threshold [45]. As a group, all pure class III antiarrhythmics increase the atrial and ventricular fibrillation threshold, decrease the ventricular defibrillation threshold, slow the rate of ventricular tachycardia, thereby preventing deterioration to ventricular fibrillation, and have the propensity to exhibit rate- or use-dependent phenomena on myocardial repolarization and refractoriness [45]. Because of their specific blocking effect on I_{Kr} channels, they inevitably prolong the QT interval Figs 5.4 and 5.5) and sometimes induce TdP. The relationship

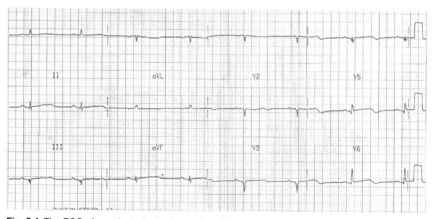

Fig. 5.4 The ECG of a patient who had a previous MI and was prescribed sotalol for nonsustained ventricular tachycardia and subsequently developed recurrent syncope. Holter recording showed frequent TdP induced by Sotalol. Note the QTc was prolonged at 710 ms.

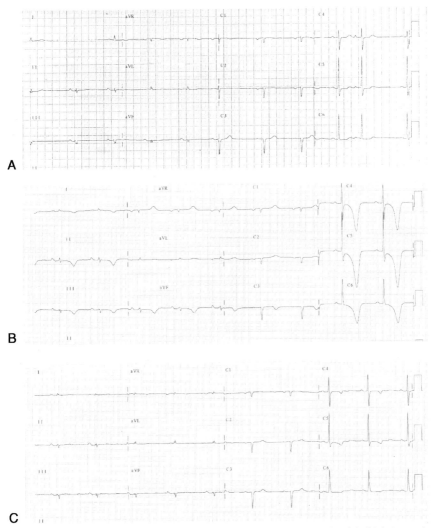

Fig. 5.5 Three ECGs from a female elderly patient: (a) before (7 years previously); (b) during and; (c) after treatment with sotalol for paroxysmal atrial fibrillation. Her coronary angiogram performed due to the appearance of her ECG during sotalol treatment was completely normal. Note the QT prolongation and deep T wave inversion during sotalol treatment in a patient with a normal QT interval but abnormal baseline repolarization and nonspecific T wave inversion. (Adapted from [6].)

between QT prolongation and plasma concentration of sotalol depends on the heart rate at which the measurements are made [47]. The incidence of proarrhythmia with d-sotalol was initially thought to be lower than its racemic counterpart because of its lesser bradycardic effect. Although some small studies supported this view and showed that d-sotalol was safe for the treatment of ventricular tachyarrhythmias [48,49], the experience from the Survival with Oral d-sotalol (SWORD) study suggested otherwise [50].

Ibutilide

Ibutilide is a methanesulfonamide derivative with a structure similar to the antiarrhythmic agent sotalol. It is available only as an intravenous agent and has been approved specially for the acute termination of atrial fibrillation and atrial flutter [51] although recent evidence showed that ibutilide is also effective in suppressing inducible monomorphic ventricular tachycardia [52].

Ibutilide is rapidly distributed to a large volume and its electrophysiologic effects dissipate rapidly after initial intravenous administration. As a result, the risk of ventricular proarrhythmic events is greatest within the first hour of administration [53,54]. The risk of TdP with ibutilide is approximately 8.3% [55], but most of this is transient and the remainder, which is sustained, is usually easily treated with intravenous magnesium, etc. Ibutilide is metabolized extensively in the liver and its metabolites are not thought to add significantly to its electrophysiologic effects [56]. Co-administration of beta-blockers or calcium-channel antagonists can induce bradycardia and increases the risk of ibutilide-induced TdP [56]. Ibutilide exerts its effect by activating the slow inward sodium ion current and blocking outward delayed rectifier I_{Kr} current, thus prolonging the action potential duration in both atria and ventricles [57–59]. At high doses, ibutilide "activates" I_{Kr}. This results in a theoretical bell-shaped activity curve, i.e., only intermediate doses are associated with prolongation of the action potential. Ibutilide increases action potential duration without significant reverse use-dependence [60] and at clinical doses increases the QT interval in a dose-related manner.

Azimilide

Azimilide, a chlorophenylfuranyl compound, is structurally different from other pure class III agents, because it lacks the methanesulfonamide. Previous attempts in developing methanesulfonamide antiarrhythmic drugs encountered two main disadvantages: namely the proarrhythmic effects of these compounds, especially during bradyarrhythmias and hypokalemia, and the decreased efficacy at higher heart rates (reverse use/rate-dependence). Thus, the development of azimilide which inhibits both I_{Ks} and I_{Kr} channels, in contrast to pure I_{Kr} blocker, may not have these disadvantages [61]. Indeed, the potassium-channel blockade induced by azimilide is not rate dependent in both atrial and ventricular tissue [62].

Azimilide was developed to prolong the time to recurrence of atrial fibrillation or flutter and paroxysmal supraventricular tachycardia. Oral azimilide at doses up to 200 mg/day prolongs the QTc interval by 4–42% [63]. The long-term safety and efficacy of azimilide is now being evaluated for the treatment of both supraventricular and ventricular arrhythmias (ASAP) [64]. The efficacy of the drug in preventing sudden cardiac death has recently been evaluated in the AzimiLide post-Infarction surVival

Evaluation (ALIVE) study. Azimilide was not associated with a reduction of mortality, but some cases of TdP were reported in association with azimilide use, usually when bradycardia, pauses and/or hypokalemia were present. The ALIVE study showed that azimilide prescribed at 100 mg has a low incidence of TdP even in high-risk postmyocardial infarction patients with reduced heart rate variability.

Tedisamil

Tedisamil, a blocker of the early rapid repolarizing I_{to} channel and I_{Kr} channel, is different from pure class III antiarrhythmic drugs because it blocks a complex aggregate of repolarizing myocardial ionic currents and has bradycardic and anti-ischaemic properties. In humans, intravenous tedisamil (0.3 mg/kg) reduces heart rate by 12% with a parallel prolongation of QTc interval (+10%) and left ventricular monophasic action potential (+16% at 90% repolarization) [65]. The QT prolonging effect diminished with increased atrial pacing rate indicating a reverse use-dependent prolongation effect [66].

In a study on isolated rabbit heart, tedisamil reduced the incidence of ventricular fibrillation compared with the control [67]. While the mechanism responsible for the antifibrillatory action of tedisamil involves blockade of I_{to} and I_{Kr} channels, it is possible that it also involves inhibition of the K_{ATP} channel in myocardial tissue [67]. While tedisamil may have multiple antiarrhythmic effects of clinical importance, there have been few clinical data in human arrhythmia. Tedisamil may be an effective agent for the termination or prevention of atrial fibrillation, but its clinical use will depend on the frequency of TdP associated with its administration.

Ersentilide

Ersentilide is a benzamide derivative, and has been found to be an effective antiarrhythmic against epinephrine-induced ventricular arrhythmias during halothane anesthesia and against ventricular arrhythmias induced by programmed electrical stimulation 3–8 days after myocardial infarction [68]. Ersentilide is an I_{Kr} and a selective β1-adrenoceptor blocker. Ersentilide prolongs the action potential duration in a reverse-use dependent manner, the effective refractory period and the duration of calcium-dependent slow response action potentials [69]. In intact dogs, ersentilide increased the magnitude of digitalis-induced delayed after-depolarizations but it neither increased nor suppressed the incidence of digitalis-induced arrhythmias [69]. Currently, the data are still lacking and until more information is available, the efficacy of ersentilide as an antiarrhythmic and its pro-arrhythmic risk cannot yet be certain.

Dofetilide

Dofetilide is a highly selective I_{Kr} blocker and increases the repolarization and refractoriness in both atrial and ventricular tissue (predominantly atrial). It is well absorbed when given orally with a good bioavailability of >90% and an elimination half-life from plasma of 7–13 h [70]. Dofetilide has a reverse use-dependent effect [71] and, at slow rates, has the propensity to cause a large increase in the QT interval of up to 200 ms after intravenous administration [72]. Dofetilide suppresses or slows inducible ventricular tachycardia in approximately 40% of patients who had been previously unsuccessfully treated with other antiarrhythmic drugs [73].

Although the Danish Investigation of Arrhythmias and Mortality ON Dofetilide-Myocardial infarction and -Congestive Heart Failure (DIAMOND-MI and -CHF) trials showed a relatively high incidence of TdP in patients with left ventricular ejection fraction ≤35% after myocardial infarction or heart failure, a detailed analysis of the study showed that the neutral mortality result in DIAMOND resulted from in-patient initiation of dofetilide [74]. If the patients developed nonfatal TdP or significant QT prolongation, dofetilide treatment was abandoned, but patients were followed in the trial on an intention-to-treat basis. This aspect of the protocol eliminated patients with high-risk proarrhythmic potential and probably prevented their subsequent death at some point during the trial follow-up. Nevertheless, the overall incidence of TdP on dofetilide was 2.1% (32 patients) among the 1511 patients that received dofetilide from both DIAMOND-MI and -CHF combined. Interestingly, the incidence of TdP with dofetilide was related to New York Heart Association functional class at baseline and not to left ventricular ejection fraction. When renal failure was present dofetilide accumulated and TdP risk increased.

Trecetilide

Trecetilide is an ibutilide analog with fluorine substitutes on the heptyl side chain [75]. It is an S-enantiomer and generally has less proarrhythmic activity than the corresponding racemates. It had excellent antiarrhythmic activity and metabolic stability and was devoid of proarrhythmic activity in the rabbit model. It retained the ability to increase the refractoriness of cardiac tissue at both slow and fast pacing rates. The drug is being developed as an antiarrhythmic drug for both oral and intravenous administration and may specifically be of value for the termination of atrial fibrillation and flutter. Unlike ibutilide, trecetilide has good oral bioavailability.

Dronedarone

Dronedarone has multiple actions (all four Vaughan-Williams classes) on the cardiac myocyte membrane, similar to amiodarone but more potent and lacks the iodine subgroup and phospholipase inhibition [40]. Dronedarone is currently under development for oral use for the treatment of a spectrum of arrhythmias including atrial fibrillation/flutter, supraventricular tachycardia, ventricular arrhythmias and the prevention of sudden cardiac death. Intravenous dronedarone suppressed early after-depolarizations, ventricular premature beats and TdP by a reduction and homogenization of repolarization of the left ventricle. In contrast to oral treatment, intravenous dronedarone shortened the ventricular repolarization parameters, resulting in suppression of early after-depolarization-dependent acquired TdP [76]. Long-term oral dronedarone increases the QT interval. A major randomized trial of dronedarone versus placebo in patients with atrial fibrillation and congestive heart failure (ANDROMEDA) was stopped prematurely because of increased mortality associated with dronedarone. The increased mortality was associated with cardiac and renal failure but not with TdP. Two large studies (EURIDES and ADONIS) in atrial fibrillation demonstrated that dronedarone reduced the recurrence of the arrhythmia by 10–20%.

Almokalant

Almokalant selectively blocks the I_{Kr} current with no significant effect on I_{Ks} current. In an animal study, almokalant prolonged the QT interval, the atrial and ventricular effective refractory periods and ventricular MAP [77]. In patients with atrial fibrillation, intravenous almokalant induced TdP in 6% of the patients [78]. The risk factors for development of TdP are female gender, ventricular extrasystoles, diuretic treatment and appearance of ECG abnormality during infusion (e.g., sequential bilateral bundle branch block, ventricular bigeminy, biphasic T wave). Patients developing TdP during almokalant infusion exhibited early pronounced QT prolongation and marked morphological T wave changes [78].

Mechanism for reducing proarrhythmic properties of antiarrhythmic drug

There are several potential mechanisms for reducing the risk of TdP with antiarrhythmic drugs, particularly class III antiarrhythmic agents. It has been suggested that prolongation of phase 2 repolarization, by augmenting the I_{Na} current, rather than phase 3 of repolarization, may help reduce the propensity to induce early after-depolarization, hence, TdP [79]. The cardiac membrane is relatively inexcitable during phase 2 compared with phase 3, which is the phase prolonged by most class III antiarrhythmic drugs thus allowing a longer interval for the development of early after-depolarizations. The blockade of the calcium channel may also diminish the induction of early after-depolarization, a property of amiodarone that may account for its low risk of TdP. An ability to diminish or eliminate the dispersion of repolarization may also be important. Generally, class III atiarrhythmic drugs have greater effect in prolonging the action potential duration and inducing early after-depolarization in Purkinje fibers and M cells compared with ventricular cells, which can lead to a greater dispersion of repolarization and potential for proarrhythmia [80,81]. An antiarrhythmic drug, such as amiodarone, that has a more homogeneous effect on Purkinje fibers and M cells may be less proarrhythmic [79]. Last but not least, an antiarrhythmic drug that produces use-dependency prolongation of action potential duration, with minimal effect at physiological heart rate and maximal effect during a rapid tachycardia may also reduce the risk of TdP. Recently antiarrhythmic agents that block the ultra-rapid potassium current (I_{kur}) have been developed. I_{kur} is expressed in the human atrium but not ventricle. These drugs may suppress atrial arrhythmias without risking QT prolongation and TdP.

The ideal antiarrhythmic drug needs to be inexpensive, effective, and above all, safe with low risk of proarrhythmia. Developers of newer antiarrhythmic agents have focused on identifying antiarrhythmic medications with the following characteristics: appropriate modification of the arrhythmia substrate, suppression of arrhythmia triggers, efficacy in pathological tissues and states, positive rate dependency, appropriate pharmacokinetics, equally effective oral and parenteral formulations, similar efficacy in arrhythmias and their surrogates, few side-effects, positive frequency-blocking actions, and a cardiac-selective ion channel blockade [2]. However, such a drug does not exist and none of the current drugs has met all of these requirements.

Conclusion

The goal of developing an antiarrhythmic drug that is effective against most arrhythmias while having a low side-effect profile, particularly in regards to proarrhythmia, remains elusive. The discordance between QT prolongation and the incidence of TdP among antiarrhythmic drugs that prolong ventricular refractoriness has stimulated immense interest in separating the salutary therapeutic effects from the adverse proarrhythmic effects of antiarrhythmic drugs. The rapidly expanding knowledge of ion channel kinetics and structure, and the molecular and genetic lesions involved in arrhythmogenesis in conditions such as the congenital long QT syndrome has helped in the understanding of the proarrhythmic mechanism of antiarrhythmic drugs. It is hoped that the availability of molecular clones that encode many of the ion channels in the human heart will help in the development of selective/lesion-specific antiarrhythmic drugs with specific profiles of channel-blocking properties that have an effective antiarrhythmic effect but with minimal proarrhythmic potential. Alternatively drugs which do not rely on blocking ion channels may be more effective and unlikely to induce TdP.

References

1 Camm AJ, Yap YG. What should we expect from the next generation of antiarrhythmic drugs? *J Cardiovasc Electrophysiol* 1999; 10: 307–17.

2 Yap YG, Camm AJ. Acquired long QT syndrome by antiarrhythmic drugs In: Oto, A, ed. *Myocardial Repolarization: From gene to Bedside*. New York: Futura, pp. 305–324, 2001.

3 Po SS, Wang DW, Yang IC, Johnson JP Jr, Nie L, Bennett PB. Modulation of HERG potassium channels by extracelluler magnesium and quinidine. *J Cardiovas Pharmacol* 1999; 33 (2): 181–5.

4 Seizer A, Wray HW. Paroxysmal ventricular fibrillation occurring during treatment of chronic atrial arrhythmias. *Circulation* 1964; 30: 17–26.

5 Jackman WM, Friday KJ, Anderson JL, Aliot EM, Clark M, Lazzara R. The long QT syndrome. A critical review, new clinical observations and a unifying hypothesis. *Prog Cardiovasc Dis* 1988; 31: 115–72.

6 Lazarra R. Antiarrhythmic drugs and torsades de pointes. *Eur Heart J* 1993; 14: H88–92.

7 Roden DM, Woosley RL, Primm RK. Incidence and clinical features of the quinidine–associated long QT syndrome: implication for patient care. *Am Heart J* 1986; 111: 1088–93.

8 Bauman JL, Bauernfeind RA, Hoff JV, Strasberg B, Swiryn S, Rosen KM. Torsades de pointes due to quinidine: observations in 31 patients. *Am Heart J* 1984; 107: 425–30.

9 Morganroth J, Horowitz LN. Incidence of proarrhythmic effects from quinidine in the outpatient treatment of benign or potentially lethal ventricular arrhythmia. *Am J Cardiol* 1985; 56: 585–7.

10 Faber TS, Zehender M, Just H. Drug-induced torsades de pointes. *Drug Safety* 1994; 11 (6): 463–76.

11 Keren A, Tzivoni D, Gavish D, Levi J, Gottlieb S, Benhorn J, Stern S. Etiology, warning signs and therapy of torsades de pointes. A study of 10 patients. *Circulation* 1981; 64: 1167–74.

12 Hewett K, Gessman L, Roden MR. Effects of procainamide, quinidine and ethmozine on delayed after depolarization. *Eur J Pharmacol* 1983; 96: 21–8.

13 Webb CL, Dick M, Rocchini AP *et al*. Quinidine syncope in children. *J Am Coll Cardiol* 1987; 9 (5): 1031–7.

14 Hohnloser SH, van de Loo A, Baedeker F. Efficacy and proarrhythmic hazards of pharmacologic cardioversion of atrial fibrillation: prospective comparison of sotalol versus quinine. *J Am Coll Cardiol* 1995; 26 (4): 825–8.

15 Piergies AA, Ruo TI, Jansyn EM, Belknap SM, Atkinson AJ Jr. Effect kinetics of N-acetylprocainamide-induced QT interval prolongation. *Clin Pharmacol Ther* 1987; 42 (1): 107–12.

16 Stevenson WG, Weiss J. Torsades de pointes due to n-acetylprocainamide. *Pacing Clin Electrophysiol* 1985; 8 (4): 528–31.

17 Vlasses PH, Ferguson RK, Rocci ML Jr, Raja RM, Porter RS, Greenspan AM. Lethal accumulation of procainamide metabolite in severe renal insufficiency. *Am J Nephrol* 1986; 6 (2): 112–6.

18 Reiter MJ, Higgins SL, Payne AG, Mann DE. Effects of quinidine versus procainamide on the. *QT Interval Am J Cardiol* 1986; 58: 512–6.

19 Lee WK, Strong JM, Kehoe RF, Dutcher JS, Atkinson AJ Jr. Antiarrhythmic efficacy of N-acetylprocainamide in patients with premature ventricular contractions. *Clin Pharmacol Ther* 1976; 19 (5 Part 1): 508–14.

20 Brosch SF, Studenik C, Heistracher P. Abolition of drug-induced early afterdepolarizations by potassium channel activators in guinea-pig Purkinje fibres. *Clin Exp Pharmacol Physiol* 1998; 25: 225–30.

21 Tzivoni D, Keren A, Stern S, Gottlieb S. Disopyramide-induced Torsade de Pointes. *Arch Intern Med* 1981; 141 (7): 946–7.

22 Nicholson WJ, Martin CE, Gracey JG, Knoch HR. Disopyramide-induced ventricular fibrillation. *Am J Cardiol* 1979; 43 (5): 1053–5.

23 Wald RW, Waxman MB, Colman JM. Torsade de pointes ventricular tachycardia. A complication of disopyramide shared with quinidine. *J Electrocardiol* 1981; 14 (3): 301–7.

24 Baker BJ, Gammill J, Massengill J, Schubert E, Karin A, Doherty JE. Concurrent use of quinidine and disopyramide: evaluation of serum concentrations and electrocardiographic effects. *Am Heart J* 1983; 105: 12–5.

25 Hulting J, Jansson B. Antiarrhythmic and electrocardiographic effects of single oral doses of disopyramide. *Eur J Clin Pharmacol* 1977; 11 (2): 91–9.

26 Minardo JD, Heger JJ, Miles WM, Zipes DP, Prystowsky EN. Clinical characteristics of patients with ventricular fibrillation during antiarrhythmic drug therapy. *N Engl J Med* 1988; 319 (5): 257–62.

27 Desai JM, Scheinman MM, Hirschfeld D, Gonzalez R, Peters RW. Cardiovascular collapse associated with disopyramide therapy. *Chest* 1981; 79 (5): 545–51.

28 Lo KS, Gantz KB, Stetson PL, Lucchesi BR, Pitt B. Disopyramide-induced ventricular tachycardia. *Arch Intern Med* 1980; 140 (3): 413–4.

29 Kaul U, Mohan JC, Narula J, Nath CS, Bhatia ML. Ajmaline-induced torsade de pointes. *Cardiology* 1985; 72 (3): 140–3.

30 Bouffard Y, Roux H, Perrot D et al. Acute ajmaline poisoning. Study of 7 cases. *Arch Mal Coeur Vaiss* 1983; 76 (7): 771–7.

31 Perrot B, Faivre G. Danger of sinoatrial block and the use of antiarrhythmic agents in myocardial infarcts. *Arch Mal Coeur Vaiss* 1982; 75 (9): 1039–48.

32 Padrini R, Piovan D, Javarnaro A, Cucchini F, Ferrari M. Pharmacokinetics and electrophysiological effects of intravenous ajmaline. *Clin Pharmacokinet* 1993; 25 (5): 408–14.

33 Enomoto K, Imoto M, Nagashima R et al. Y. Effects of ajmaline on nonsodium ionic currents in guinea pig ventricular myocytes. *Jpn Heart J* 1995; 36 (4): 465–76.

34 Hondeghem LM, Snyder DJ. Class III antiarrhythmic agents have a lot of potential but a long way to go: reduced effectiveness and danger of reverse use dependence. *Circulation* 1990; 81: 686–90.

35 Singh BN. Antiarrhythmic actions of amiodarone: a profile of a paradoxical agent. *Am J Cardiol* 1996; 78 (Suppl. 4A): 41–53.

36 Hohnloser SH, Klingenheben T, Singh BN. Amiodarone-associated proarrhythmic effects. A review with special reference to torsades de pointes tachycardia. *Ann Intern Med* 1994; 121: 529–35.

37 Scheinman MM, Levine JH, Cannom DS et al. Dose-ranging study of intravenous amiodarone in patients with life-threatening ventricular tachyarrhythmias. The Intravenous Amiodarone Multicenter Investigators Group. *Circulation* 1995; 92: 3264–72.

38 Amiodarone Trials Meta-analysis. Effect of prophylactic amiodarone on mortality after acute myocardial infarction and in congestive heart failure: meta-analysis of individual data from 6500 patients in randomised trials. *Lancet* 1997; 350: 1417–24.

39 Kodama I, Kamiya K, Toyama J. Cellular electropharmacology of amiodarone. *Cardiovasc Res* 1997; 35 (1): 13–29.

40 Sun W, Sarma Jonnalagedda SMS, Singh B. Electrophysiological effects of dronedarone (SR33589), a noniodinated benzofuran derivative, in the rabbit heart. Comparison with amiodarone. *Circulation* 1999; 100: 2276–81.

41 Sanguinetti MC. Modulation of potassium channels by antiarrhythmic and antihypertensive drugs. *Hypertension* 1992; 19: 228–36.

42 Funck-Brentano C. Pharmacokinetic and pharmacodynamic profiles of d-sotalol and d,l-sotalol. *Eur Heart J* 1993; 14 (Suppl. H): 30–5.

43 Hohnloser SH, Zabel M, van de Loo A, Klingenheben T, Just H. Efficacy and safety of sotalol in patients with complex ventricular arrhythmias. *Int J Cardiol* 1992; 37 (3): 283–91.

44 Hohnloser SH. Proarrhythmia with class III antiarrhythmic drugs: types, risks, and management. *Am J Cardiol* 1997; 80 (8A): 82G–89G.

45 MacNeil DJ, Davies RO, Deitchman D. Clinical safety profile of sotalol in the treatment of arrhythmas. *Am J Cardiol* 1993; 72: 44A–50A.

46 Kuhlkamp V, Mermi J, Mewis C, Seipel L. Efficacy and proarrhythmia with the use of d,l-sotalol for sustained ventricular tachyarrhythmias. *J Cardiovasc Pharmacol* 1997; 29 (3): 373–81.

47 Funck-Brentano C, Kibleur Y, Le Coz F, Poirier JM, Mallet A, Jaillon P. Rate dependence of sotalol-induced prolongation of ventricular repolarization during exercise in humans. *Circulation* 1991; 83 (2): 536–45.

48 Brachmann J, Schols W, Beyer T, Montero M, Enders B, Kubler W. Acute and chronic antiarrhythmic efficacy of d-sotalol in patients with sustained ventricular tachyarrhythmias. *Eur Heart J* 1993; 14 (Suppl.): H85–H87.

49 Koch KT, Duren DR, van Zwieten PA. Long-term antiarrhythmic efficacy and safety of d-sotalol in patients with ventricular tachycardia and a low ejection fraction. *Cardiovasc Drugs Ther* 1995; 9 (3): 437–43.

50 Waldo AL, Camm AJ, deRuyter H *et al*. Effect of d-sotalol on mortality in patients with left ventricular dysfunction after recent and remote myocardial infarction. *Lancet* 1996; 348: 7–12.

51 Ellenbogen KA, Clemo HF, Stambler BS, Wood MA, Vander Lugt JT. Efficacy of ibutilide for termination of atrial fibrillation and flutter. *Am J Cardiol* 1996; 78 (Suppl.): 42–5.

52 Wood MA, Stambler BS, Ellenbogen KA *et al*. Suppression of inducible ventricular tachycardia by ibutilide in patients with coronary artery disease. *Am Heart J* 1998; 135: 1048–54.

53 Naccarelli GV, Lee KS, Gibson JK, Vander Lugt J. Electrophysiology and pharmacology of ibutilide. *Am J Cardiol* 1996; 78 (Suppl.): 12–6.

54 Kowey PR, Vander Lugt JT, Luderer JR. Safety and risk/benefit analysis of ibutilide for acute conversion of atrial fibrillation/flutter. *Am J Cardiol* 1996; 78 (Suppl.): 46–52.

55 Stambler BS, Wood M, Ellenbogen KA, Perry KT, Wakefield LK, VanderLugt JT and the Ibutilide Repeat Dose Study Investigators. *Circulation* 1996; 94: 1613–21.

56 Kowey PR, Marichak RA, Rials SJ, Bharucha D. Pharmacologic and pharmacokinetic profile of class III antiarrhythmic drugs. *Am J Cardiol* 1997; 80 (8A): 16G–23G.

57 Lee KS. Ibutilide, a new compound with potent class III antiarrhythmic activity, activates a slow inward Na current in guinea pig ventricular cells. *J Pharmacol Exp Ther* 1992; 262: 99–108.

58 Lee KS, Lee EW. Ionic mechanism of ibutilide in human atrium: evidence for a drug-induced Na+ current through a nifedipine inhibited inward channel. *J Pharmacol Exp Ther* 1998; 286: 9–22.

59 Yang T, Snyders DJ, Roden DM. Ibutilide, a methanesulfonanilide antiarrhythmic, is a potent blocker of the rapidly activating delayed rectifier K current (IKr) in AT-1 cells. *Circulation* 1995; 91: 216–21.

60 Buchanan LV, LeMay RJ, Gibson JK. Comparison of the class III agent dl-sotalol HCl and ibutilide fumerate for atrial reverse use dependence and antiarrhythmic effects. *PACE* 1996: 19 (Abstract): 687.

61 Fermini B, Jurkiewicz NK, Jow B. Use-dependent effect of the class III antiarrhythmic agent NE-10064 (azimilide) on cardiac repolarization: block of delayed rectifier and l-type calcium currents. *J Cardiovasc Pharmacol* 1995; 26: 259–71.

62 Busch AE, Eigenberger B, Jurkiewicz NK, Salata JJ, Pica A, Suessbrich H, Lang F. Blockade of HERG channels by the class III antiarrhythmic azimilide: mode of action. *Br J Pharmacol* 1998; 123: 23–30.

63 Corey AE, Al-khalidi H, Brezovic C, Marcello S, Parekh N, Taylor K, Karam R. Azimilide pharmacokinetics and pharmacodynamics upon multiple oral dosing. *Clin Pharmacol Ther* 1997; 61: 205.

64 Karam R, Marcello S, Brooks RR, Corey AE, Moore A. Azimilide dihydrochloride, a novel antiarrhythmic agent. *Am J Cardiol* 1998; 81 (6A): 40D–46D.

65 Black SC, Butterfield JL, Lucchesi BR. Protection against programmed electrical stimulation-induced ventricular tachycardia and sudden cardiac death by NE-10064, a class III antiarrhythmic drug. *J Cardiovasc Pharmacol* 1993; 22: 810–8.

66 Bargheer K, Bode F, Klein HU, Trappe HJ, Franz MR, Lichtlen PR. Prolongation of monophasic action potential duration and the refractory period in the human heart by tedisamil, a new potassium-blocking agent. *Eur Heart J* 1994; 15: 1409–14.

67 Chi L, Park JL, Friedrichs GS, Banglawala YA, Perez MA, Tanhehco EJ, Lucchesi BR. Effects of tedisamil (KC-8857) on cardiac electrophysiology and ventricular fibrillation in the rabbit isolated heart. *Br J Pharmacol* 1996; 117: 1261–9.

68 Argentieri TM, Troy HH, Carroll MS, Doroshuk CM, Sullivan ME. Electrophysiologic activity and antiarrhythmic efficacy of CK-3579, a new antiarrhythmic agent with β-adrenergic blocking properties. *J Cardiovasc Pharmacol* 1992; 21: 647.

69 Lee JH, Rosenshtraukh L, Beloshapko G, Rosen MR. The electrophysiologic effects of ersentilide on canine hearts. *Eur J Pharmacol* 1995; 285: 25–35.

70 Tham TCK, MacLennan BA, Harron DGW. Pharmacodynamics and pharmacokinetics of the novel class III antiarrhythmic drug UK-68,798 in man. *Br J Clin Pharmacol* 1991; 31 (II): 243–9.

71 Sedgwick M, Rasmussen HS, Walker D, Cobbe SM. Pharmacokinetic and pharmacodynamic effect of UK-68,798. A new potential class III antiarrhythmic drug. *Br J Pharmacol* 1991; 31: 515–9.

72 Rasmussen HS, Allen MJ, Blackburn KJ, Butrous GS, Dalrymple HW. Dofetilide, a novel class III antiarrhythmic agent. *J Cardiovasc Pharmacol* 1992; 20 (Suppl. 2): S96–S105.

73 Bashir Y, Thomsen PEB, Kingma JH *et al.* Electrophysiologic profile and efficacy of intravenous dofetilide (UK-68,798), a new class III antiarrhythmic drug, in patients with sustained monomorphic ventricular tachycardia. *Am J Cardiol* 1995; 76: 1040–4.

74 Torp-Pedersen C, Moller M, Bloch-Thomsen PE *et al.* Dofetilide in patients with congestive heart failure and left ventricular dysfunction. Danish Investigations of Arrhythmia and Mortality on Dofetilide Study Group. *N Engl J Med* 1999; 341 (12): 857–65.

75 Hester JB, Gibson JK, Buchanan LV *et al.* Progress toward the development of a safe and effective agent for treating reentrant cardiac arrhythmias: synthesis and evaluation of ibutilide analogs with enhanced metabolic stability and diminished proarrhythmic potential. *J Med Chem* 2001; 44 (7): 1099–115.

76 Verduyn SC, Vos MA, Leunissen HD, van Opstal JM, Wellens HJ. Evaluation of the acute electrophysiologic effects of intravenous dronedarone, an amiodarone-like agent, with special emphasis on ventricular repolarization and acquired torsade de pointes arrhythmias. *J Cardiovasc Pharmacol* 1999; 33 (2): 212–22.

77 Duker G, Almgren O, Carlsson L. Electrophysiologic and hemodynamic effects of H234/09 (almokalant), quinidine, and (+) -sotalol in anesthesized dog. *J Cardiovasc Pharmacol* 1992; 20: 458–65.

78 Houltz B, Darpo B, Edvardsson N *et al.* Electrocardiographic and clinical predictors of torsades de pointes induced by almokalant infusion in patients with chronic atrial fibrillation or flutter: a prospective study. *Pacing Clin Electrophysiol* 1998; 21 (5): 1044–57.

79 Nair LA, Grant AO. Emerging class III antiarrhythmic agents: mechanism of action and proarrhythmic potential. *Cardiovasc Drug Ther* 1997; 11: 149–67.

80 Li ZY, Maldonado C, Zee-Cheng C, Hiromasa S, Kupersmith J. Purkinje fiber–papillary muscle interaction in the genesis of triggered activity in guinea pig model. *Cardiovasc Res* 1992; 26: 543 –8.

81 Antzelevitch C, Sicouri S. Clinical relevance of cardiac arrhythmias generated by afterdepolarization. The role of M cell in the generation of U wave, triggered activity and torsades de pointes. *J Am Coll Cardiol* 1994; 23: 259–77.

CHAPTER 6

Risk of QT prolongation and torsades de pointes with antihistamines

Introduction

Antihistamines (H_1-receptor antagonists) are one of the most frequently prescribed drugs worldwide for the treatment of allergic conditions such as seasonal allergic rhinitis, particularly in the developed countries. The use of first generation antihistamines, such as diphenhydramine, hydroxyzine, chlorpheniramine, brompheniramine and cyproheptadine is limited by their anticholinergic and sedative properties which has been described to occur in more than 50% of patients receiving therapeutic dosages. Serious adverse events are unusual following overdoses of first generation antihistamines although life-threatening adverse events have been described. When the so-called "second generation" antihistamines terfenadine and astemizole were introduced, they were widely embraced and quickly used by clinicians since their effectiveness was equal to the first generation antihistamines in relieving symptoms associated with hyperhistaminic conditions, without the soporific effects of the first generation agents. Unfortunately, since 1990, after approximately 10 years of widespread clinical use, both terfenadine and astemizole have been reported to cause QT prolongation and, in some cases, TdP and sudden death [1–12]. In some cases of proarrhythmia, it is due to an overdose of the drugs, i.e., at doses exceeding that recommended by the manufacturer [1,3,4,5,6,7,9] although not exclusively [2,8,10–12]. In other cases, the cardiotoxicity of terfenadine or astemizole was noted at normal dosage but with concurrent use of other drugs that inhibit cytochrome P450 CYP3A4 drug metabolism (e.g., azole antifungals and macrolide antibiotics), in patients with impaired liver function [9], congenital long QT syndrome [8,10,12] or coadministration with drugs that prolong the QT interval by the same or other mechanism (e.g., antiarrhythmics, antipsychotics, tricyclic antidepressants) [11,12].

   As a result of these adverse reports, terfenadine and astemizole have since been suspended in several European countries and by the Food and Drug Administration (FDA) in the USA. The potential life-threatening cardiotoxicities of the second generation antihistamines led to the search for noncardiotoxic and nonsedating agents. Loratadine, fexofenadine, mizolastine, ebastine, azelastine, cetirizine and acrivastine are the first of the new third generation antihistamines. However, the occurrence of cardiotoxic effects in some patients taking terfenadine and astemizole has led to the speculation that other nonsedating antihistamines may induce similar cardiotoxic effects. The evidence, however, suggests that the adverse cardiac potential may not be a class property of nonsedating antihistamines, as will be discussed below. The cardiac safety profile of the H_1-antihistamines marketed in EEC countries is now being monitored by the European health authorities.

Properties of antihistamines determining the proarrhythmic toxicity

The association of nonsedating antihistamines and TdP has been reported mainly with terfenadine and astemizole. Some antihistamines exhibit their cardiac effects at therapeutic histamine-receptor-blocking concentration, whereas others show cardiac effects at supra-therapeutic concentration or have not shown any significant cardiac effects. There are several factors that may be responsible for the varying cardiac action of antihistamines.

Potassium ion-channel blockade

Like class III antiarrhythmics, terfenadine and astemizole prolong the monophasic action potential and QT interval, which leads to the development of early after-depolarizations and TdP through inhibition of I_{Kr} channels [13–15]. Not all nonsedating antihistamines block the I_{Kr} channels to the same degree (Fig. 6.1). Among the antihistamines evaluated, astemizole, terfenadine and ebastine have shown blocking effects in I_{Kr} channels expressed in *Xenopus* oocytes [16–18]. Mizolastine also blocks I_{Kr} channels in Chinese hamster ovarian cells although in a reversible manner and at concentrations significantly higher than those corresponding to therapeutic free plasma

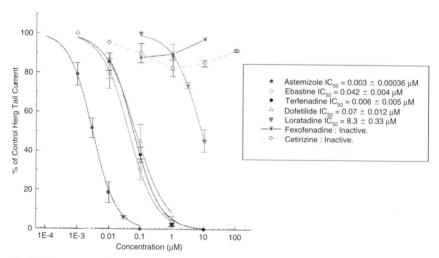

Fig. 6.1 Percentage of I_{Kr} current available vs. the concentration of nonsedating antihistamines.

levels. Terfenadine and ebastine [16], but not mizolastine [19], can also block the slow delayed rectifier I_{Ks} channel in guinea-pig dissociated ventricular myocytes. Loratadine does not block cloned I_{Kr} channels expressed in *Xenopus* oocytes (up to 10 μm), and in guinea-pig ventricular myocytes (up to 3 μm), whereas in higher concentration, it can block both heterogeneously and constitutively expressed I_{Kr} channels [20–22]. In other words, in I_{Kr} potassium channels expressed in either *Xenopus* oocytes or human neuroblastoma cells, loratadine at a concentration of 30 m produced a blockade of 20–30%, whereas the corresponding values for terfenadine and astemizole were about 80–100% [21].

In contrast, cetirizine, despite having similar antihistaminic potency *in vivo* with respect to other antihistamines, does not block the I_{Kr} channel in heterogeneously expressed *Xenopus* oocytes (up to 30 μm) or prolong ventricular repolarization at the highest therapeutic level in a canine model of long QT syndrome [21,23]. Similarly, fexofenadine, the carboxylate metabolite of terfenadine, has no I_{Kr}-blocking effect, even at a concentration 30 times greater than the concentration of terfenadine producing half-maximal effect [24,25].

Thus, there are significant differences in the ability of antihistamines in blocking the different members of the cardiac potassium-channel family. It appears that those antihistamines such as terfenadine that suppress simultaneously more than one channel involved in the lengthening of the action potential (i.e., I_{Kr} and I_{Ks}) and which block I_{Kr} at low concentration possess higher propensity to induce arrhythmias, whereas nonsedating antihistamines, which do not block the I_{Kr} channels (e.g., fexofenadine, cetirizine) or block the channel with lower potency (e.g., loratidine) should be less cardiotoxic.

Physico-chemical properties

Other drug-related factors such as the physico-chemical properties of the antihistamines (e.g., diarylalkylamine moiety, quaternization of diphenhydramine, lipophilicity of the side chain) and its metabolic profile (e.g., tissue distribution) may also contribute to the cardiac toxicity of antihistamines. Like class III antiarrhythmic agents, certain antihistamines possess a diarylalkylamine moiety, which is believed to inhibit the potassium channels [13]. Quaternization of diphenhydramine can result in a potent class I antiarrhythmic agent with long duration of action and notable tachycardia [13]. Lipophilicity of the side chain (nitrogen substitution) is also important in the potassium-channel blocking activities of antihistamines [13]. In this aspect, mizolastine is less lipophilic compared with most of the antihistamines (loratidine, astemizole, ebastine, terfenadine) and does not contain either diarylakylamine nor diphenhydramine moieties. A low lipophilicity is reflected in a small volume of distribution, both characteristics being considered important for the cardiac safety profile of an antihistamine drug [26]. In addition, there are major differences in tissue distribution and myocardial fixation among H_1-antihistamines. A low apparent volume of distribution seems to be associated with low tissue fixation (i.e., tissue levels lower than blood levels). For instance, heart/plasma ratios in animals are 4 in rats for terfenadine [27], 400 in dogs for astermizole [28,29], but only 0.5 for mizolastine in guinea-pigs (unpublished data).

Hepatic metabolism

Most but not all of the nonsedating antihistamines are metabolized via the hepatic cytochrome P450 CYP3A4 system (Table 6.1). Therefore, administration of these antihistamines in patients with compromised liver function or concomitant administration of drugs (e.g., imidazole antifungals, macrolide antibiotics) (Table 6.2) or food (e.g., grapefruit juice) that inhibit the hepatic cytochrome P450 CYP3A4 may result in the accumulation of the parent drug and cardiotoxicity [11]. For instance, terfenadine undergoes rapid first-pass metabolism by cytochrome P450 CYP3A4 hepatic enzymes and is transformed into its active metabolite terfenadine cardoxylate which has no effect on the I_{Kr} potassium channel, even at high concentration [12]. However, inhibition of the hepatic oxidative metabolism of terfenadine by macrolide antibiotics (erythromycin, clarithromycin) or imidazole antifungals (e.g., ketoconazole, itraconazole) will result in an accumulation and increased bioavailability of the cardiotoxic pro-drug [13,30]. In addition, drugs such as erythromycin and ketoconazole can in themselves prolong the QT interval. Concomitant administration of terfenadine and any of these antimicrobial therapies will produce marked QT prolongation that correlates with plasma concentration of unmetabolized terfenadine and increase the risk of proarrhythmia [31]. Concomitant administration of terfenadine with drugs that can inhibit metabolic activity of hepatic cytochrome P450 or those that prolong QT interval must be avoided.

In the case of astemizole, the P450 isoenzyme CYP3A4 metabolizes the drug into two active metabolites, desmethylastemizole and norastemizole. The QT prolongation is mainly caused by astemizole and desmethylastemizole [13]. Ebastine, a highly lipophilic compound, is a pro-drug, which is metabolized to a large extent through the cytochrome P450 CYP3A4 and its plasma concentration is increased after oral dosage by pretreatment with ketoconazole [32]. Mizolastine is less dependent on cytochrome P450 hepatic

Table 6.1 Nonsedating antihistamines and their major metabolic pathway.

Nonsedating antihistamines	Major metabolic pathway
Terfenadine	Hepatic P450 CYP3A4
Astemizole	Hepatic P450 CYP3A4
Ebastine	Hepatic P450 CYP3A4 & CYP2D6
Loratadine	Hepatic P450 CYP3A4 & CYP2D6
Mizolastine	Mainly via glucuronidation (65%), less on hydroxylation via hepatic P450 CYP 3A4 & 2A6
Fexofenadine	Renal
Cetirizine	60% via the renal route and 40% via the hepatic route

Table 6.2 Drugs, food and conditions that can inhibit hepatic cytochrome P450 CYP3A4 enzyme activity.

Azoles antifungals	Ketoconazole
	Miconazole
	Itraconazole
	Fluconazole
	Metronidazole
Macrolide antibiotics	Erythromycin
	Clarithromycin
	Troleandomycin
	Josamycin
	Flurythromycin
	Ponsinomycin
Antidepressant	Fluvoxamine
	Fluoxetine
	Paroxitine
	Sertraline
	Nefazodone
HIV protease inhibitors or non-nucleoside reverse transcriptase inhibitor (NNRTI)	Amprenavir
	Indinavir
	Nelfinavir
	Ritonavir
	Saquinavir
	Delavirdine (NNRTI)
Antiulcer	Ranitidine
	Cimetidine
	Omeprazole
Ethinyloestradiol	Estrogen
	Oral contraceptive
Calcium antagonists	Diltiazem
	Verapamil
	Nifedipine
Tetracyclines	Tetracycline
	Doxycycline
Antituberculosis drug	Isoniazid
Antimalarial	Primaquine
Streptogramin antibiotic	Quinupristin/dalfopristin
Quinolones antibiotic	Norfloxacin
	Ciprofloxacin
	Enoxacin
Antiarrhythmic drug	Amiodarone
	Quinidine
Antihypertensive drug	Hydralazine
Food	Grapefruit juice
	Alcohol
Other conditions	Smoking
	Liver disease
	Genetic polymorphism

metabolism than astemizole, terfenadine and ebastine. Thus, mizolastine has relatively little (1.5–50%) pharmacokinetic interactions with ketoconazole and erythromycin compared with the drugs mentioned above; the increase in mizolastine plasma concentrations, observed with systemic ketoconazole and erythromycin, led to plasma concentrations equivalent to those obtained with a 15–20 mg dose of mizolastine alone.

Cetirizine and fexofenadine differ from the other nonsedating antihistamines because they are eliminated primarily as the parent drug with little metabolism [33]. In adults, cetirizine is eliminated 60% via the renal route and 40% via the hepatic route. Patients with renal and hepatic impairment are advised to decrease the dose. Fexofenadine is eliminated primarily by the faecal route (80%) and only 10% by the renal route. In consequence, the drug interactions critical for terfenadine, for instance, are less relevant, and renal disease rather than liver disease could result in elevated plasma concentrations.

Grapefruit juice contains furanocoumarins (e.g., 6′, 7′-dihydroxybergamottin and its dimers), which are potent inhibitors of CYP3A4, as well as causing a rapid loss of enzyme activity of intestinal but not hepatic cytochrome CYP3A4. Although most studies on drug–grapefruit interactions have used double-strength grapefruit juice [34], recent evidence with terfenadine has shown significant effects with regular-strength grapefruit juice and freshly squeezed juice [33]. Therefore, grapefruit juice should be avoided when taking these drugs. Some other fruit juices also block intestinal CYP3A4.

Effects of nonsedating antihistamines on QT intervals

Currently, the potential effects of any new H_1-antihistamine on human cardiac repolarization are carefully examined during its clinical development mainly through the assessment of its potential to prolong the QT interval and the monitoring of potential cardiac events.

Terfenadine increases the QT interval in a dose-dependent manner and QT-interval prolongation has been shown to correlate with terfenadine concentration [35,36]. This effect is significantly more marked in patients with cardiovascular disease [36]. Compared to baseline, terfenadine 60 mg twice daily is associated with a QTc increase of 6 ms in normal subjects and a 12-ms increase in patients with cardiovascular disease [36]. Astemizole prolongs the QT interval but there is a lack of correlation between dose, plasma concentration and QT prolongation [13,31]. The action-potential duration-prolonging effects of both terfenadine and astemizole correspond to the reverse use-dependence phenomenon.

There has been no report of QT prolongation or ventricular arrhythmias with ebastine at therapeutic dosage or at a dosage three times the recommended dosage (60 mg/day) [31,37]. At a dosage five times the recommended dosage (100 mg/day), ebastine was reported to cause a small QT prolongation (10.3 ms and <10%) that was considered not clinically meaningful, although it was statistically significant compared with placebo [37]. However, when the very same study was analyzed using more appropriate means for heart rate correction, no QTc interval prolongation was found [38]. A detailed study showed that the minor QT prolongation with ebastine (or possibly with other drugs) is critically dependent on the precision of the rate correction formulae and influenced by the natural variability of the QTc interval. For instance, while all generalized heart rate correction formulas showed consistent QT prolongation with terfenadine, results were inconsistent with ebastine. Bazett's correction formula suggested significant QT interval increase on ebastine but correction using the Lecocq formula found a significant QT interval decrease. Even with an optimized heart rate correction formula ($QTc = QT/RR^{0.314}$) from pooled QT/RR regression during drug-free state, the minor QT prolongation with ebastine was not consistent. When using individualized heart rate correction, the QTc changes in a four-way cross-over study after a 7-day course of placebo, 60 mg of ebastine, 100 mg of ebastine and 100 mg of terfenadine were: -2.76 ± 5.51 ms, $P = 0.022$; -3.15 ± 9.17 ms, $P = $ NS; -2.61 ± 9.55 ms, $P = $ NS; 12.43 ± 15.25 ms, $P = 0.00057$, respectively [38]. In spite of using precise correction technology, this study has also shown differences between separate drug-free days of up to 4.70 ± 8.92 ms ($P = 0.017$). Similar findings have been later replicated even when using the most precise measurement technology (Malik M., 2003, unpublished observation). Hence, there is not only a circadian rhythm of the rate correct QTc interval but the duration of the QT interval also depends on cardiac autonomic input the average level of which may change day-to-day. Interpretation of small changes in the QTc interval, even when highly statistically significant, is therefore problematic. The distinction between drug effects and autonomic influence due to, for instance, psychosocial conditioning of investigated subjects, is frequently difficult if not directly impossible to make.

Loratadine had no effect on the QT interval when administered alone, at supra-therapeutic doses, or in combination with ketoconazole or erythromycin [39–41]. In one study, no patients had a QTc interval of more than 440 ms even when given at a dosage four times the recommended dosage (40 mg) during the 3 months of administration [39]. Another study also showed that when given at 10 mg dosage in healthy volunteers, concomitant use of the blockers of CYP3A4 (ketoconazole or cimetidine) triplicated and doubled the plasma concentrations of loratadine and desloratadine, respectively, with no significant change in the QT interval [42]. However, when loratadine given at 20 mg daily was coadministered with nefazodone, there was a statistically significant prolongation of the QT interval, which correlated with the plasma concentration of the former (22 ms, CI 14–30, $P < 0.05$) [43]. Desloratadine is the active metabolite of loratadine with a half-life of 21–24 h. It appears to exert no blocking effect on I_{Kr} potassium channel, and when administered either alone in a higher dose or in combination with ketoconazole or erythromycin, no prolongation of the QT interval was observed [44,45].

The clinical experience with mizolastine, particularly in potentially high-risk patients, is still limited. An overview of the QT interval monitoring performed during the clinical development of mizolastine, showed that this new selective second generation H_1-antihistamine has no significant effect on cardiac repolarization in humans [46]. Mizolastine was administered orally up to 75 mg single dose and 40 mg repeated dose in healthy volunteers (i.e., 7.5 and 4 times the recommended daily dose, respectively) and at a dose of 10 or 15 mg in patients. In healthy volunteers, there was no increased incidence of QTc value >440 ms or ΔQTc $\geq$40 ms compared with placebo. No dose-related increase in QTc interval was observed. In patients, the mean QTc interval changes from baseline were not significantly different between mizolastine and placebo. There was little or no idiosyncratic QT interval prolongation in volunteers or patients receiving mizolastine. Mizolastine did not induce changes in T/U wave morphologies in humans.

Cetirizine, the metabolite of hydroxyzine, a first generation antihistamine, which has been reported to be associated at high doses with T wave changes, did not cause QT prolongation [31]. In studies conducted in normal subjects, cetirizine at supra-therapeutic doses was also devoid of an effect on QT interval [47]. Similarly, there was no dose-related increase in QT interval or significant increase in mean QT interval with fexofenadine, the carboxylate metabolite of terfenadine, in dosage up to 240 mg, twice a day for 12 months compared with placebo [48]. Recently, extensive ECG data from more than 2100 patients receiving fexofenadine or placebo in controlled clinical trials demonstrated that fexofenadine does not increase QT interval, even when administered long term in doses 10-fold that of recommended dosage [49]. In controlled trials with approximately 6000 subjects, no case of fexofenadine-associated TdP was observed in this large series [49]. This is probably not surprising, given that fexofenadine does not block the I_{Kr} potassium channel. There has been one case report of possible fexofenadine-induced QT prolongation and ventricular arrhythmia [50] but the association is confounded by the patient's age, hypertensive hypertrophy and sudden cessation of carvedilol, which may constitute the risk factors for QT prolongation and ventricular arrhythmia. While there had been two further case reports in the literature of ventricular tachyarrhythmias associated with the use of fexofenadine (one ventricular fibrillation on a patient with pre-existing congenital long QT syndrome and the other of a patient with possible QT prolongation and life-threatening arrhythmias), the lack of detailed clinical data renders it difficult to be certain of the causal relationship between fexofenadine and the arrhythmias in these case reports. The significance of these single cases of reported cardiotoxicity with fexofenadine use remains obscure so far [51–54]. Thus, a definitive conclusion cannot be drawn from these few possible adverse cardiac effect of fexofenadine given the extensive clinical and experimental evidence that suggests that TdP should not be a risk with exposure to this drug.

Newer nonsedating antihistamines such as azelatine have no electrocardiographic effects when administered at several times the recommended dose or concomitantly with agents that inhibit their metabolism and elimination in human volunteers [55]. The data on acrivastine is currently lacking and further information on its cardiac safety is urgently needed. In one study on isolated canine cardiac Purkinje fibers at a 100-mm concentration (i.e., 10 times higher than the plasma concentrations observed in clinical studies), acrivastine caused no significant change in the duration of the action potential [56] According to the international WHO database (see below), the use of acrivastine has been related to cardiac death or arrhythmias typically caused by terfenadine.

The effect of nonsedating antihistamines that are metabolized by cytochrome P450 CYP3A4 on the QT interval is markedly increased when they are coadministered with an enzyme inhibitor. For instance, a mean of 82 ms increase in QTc interval at 12 h after dosing (i.e., at or near trough) was reported when terfenadine is coadministrated with ketoconazole [30].

In the case of loratadine, no significant changes in QTc interval from baseline (approximately 400 ms) were demonstrated when ketoconazole, erythromycin and cimetidine, respectively, were given in combination with loratadine [57–59]. Other studies disagree and report marginal QTc changes.

With mizolastine, the ECG parameters were not modified when coadministered with erythromycin, compared to the effect of each coadministrated drug alone. The minor QT interval prolongation observed during the coadministration of ketoconazole with mizolastine ($\approx +7$ ms) might be attributable to the ketoconazole itself [60]. The same explanation applied when ketoconazole (400 mg) was coadministered with cetirizine (20 mg, twice the recommended dose), which produced a minor QT prolongation of 17.4 ms compared with 9.1 ms with cetirizine alone [61].

Interaction studies showed no significant increases in QTc when fexofenadine 120 mg twice daily was administered in combination with erythromycin (500 mg three times daily) or ketoconazole (400 mg once daily) after dosing to steady state (6.5 days) [50].

Incidence of cardiac events with commonly prescribed nonsedating antihistamines

The WHO adverse-drug-reaction database provides a source of data on spontaneous adverse drug reactions from 17 countries where nonsedating antihistamines are available. Data reported includes total rate and rhythm disorders, selected reactions (QT prolongation, TdP, ventricular tachyarrhythmias, cardiac arrest and supraventricular tachycardia), cardiac and sudden deaths. Data from 1986 to 1996 reported: 106 cases of selected reactions, 13 cardiac and sudden deaths for loratadine; 19 cases of selected reactions, two cardiac and sudden deaths for cetirizine; one case of selected reaction and no incidence of cardiac and sudden death for acrivastine [62]. When calculated as reports per million defined daily doses (DDD) sold, all three antihistamines have a very low reporting rate. Specifically, the reporting rates for cardiac and sudden deaths were approximately 0.005 for loratadine and 0.0008 for cetirizine and none for acrivastine compared with 0.038 for terfenadine. Although the reported incidences of deaths were themselves very low compared with terfenadine, the type of report and analysis has attracted some criticism for potential flaws and biases [63,64]. For instance, the report does not take into account the spontaneous rate of background cardiac events in the untreated population and the inclusion of a wide variety of cardiac events in a composite numerator, rather than specific ventricular events of relevance to nonsedating antihistamines. This makes the analysis questionable [64]. Furthermore, it is important to remember that spontaneous adverse reports cannot be used to measure the true incidence of the particular event but merely give a rough idea of possible differences. The FDA, which monitors, analyzes and reviews individual reports and follow-up of cases of adverse drug reactions with antihistamines, did not find any definitive causal association between loratadine, cetirizine or acrivastine and ventricular tachyarrhythmia up to 1997.

It should be emphasized that apart from the specific contraindications described, the incidence of cardiotoxicity with antihistamines is very low in view of the widespread use of the drugs. In a cohort study carried out in the UK using the UK-based General Practice Research database on 197 425 persons who received 513 012 prescriptions between January 1, 1992 and September 30, 1996, the crude incidence of idiopathic ventricular arrhythmias with the use of antihistamines (acrivastine, astemizole, cetirizine, loratadine and terfenadine) was calculated as 1.9 per 10 000 person-years (95%CI: 1.0–3.6) and a relative risk of 4.2 (95%CI: 1.5–11.8) as compared with nonuse. Astemizole presented the highest relative risk (RR = 19.0; 95%CI: 4.8–76.0) of all study drugs, while terfenadine (RR = 2.1; 95%CI: 0.5–8.5) was in the range of other nonsedating antihistamines. Older age was associated with a greater risk of ventricular arrhythmias (RR = 7.4; 95%CI: 2.6–21.4) and seemed to increase the effect of antihistamines (RR = 6.4; 95%CI: 1.7–24.8). Thus, the use of nonsedating antihistamines increases the risk of ventricular arrhythmias by a factor of four in the general population. The absolute effect is, however, quite low requiring 57 000 prescriptions, or 5300 person-years of use for one case to occur [65]. Nevertheless, when antihistamines are widely prescribed for a self-limiting, nonfatal disease, often in children and young adults, the attributable risk must be assessed very carefully. It will also be very difficult to conduct a large controlled clinical study to examine the causal association between nonsedating antihistamines and ventricular arrhythmias. Any crude adverse event report must be used in perspective and to detect trends and generate hypotheses that may guide surveillance and help plan future studies. The European Association of Allergy and Clinical Immunology (EAACI) published a guideline on the use of nonsedating antihistamines to avoid any unwanted arrhythmogenic effect associated with their use [66].

Proarrhythmic risk of sedating antihistamines

Among the first generation sedating antihistamines, clemastine, hydroxyzine, brompheniramine, chlorpheniramine, and diphenhydramine have all elicited a dose-dependent slowing of cardiac repolarization in the isolated perfused feline heart model, as indicated by the QT prolongations in one study [67]. The concentrations of drugs tested ranged from 1 to $30\,\mu$m. Of the drugs analyzed, clemastine and hydroxyzine appeared to be the most potent (relative IC_{50} values, 5.2 and $6.6\,\mu$m, respectively), causing the QT to lengthen by as much as 40–50% at a concentration of $10\,\mu$m. Brompheniramine, chlorpheniramine, and diphenhydramine displayed intermediate potencies with respect to QT prolongation (relative IC_{50} values, 11–$13\,\mu$m), whereas cyproheptadine, chlorcyclizine, and promethazine were the least potent of the antihistamines tested (relative IC_{50} values, 16–$20\,\mu$m).

Other studies also showed that chlorpheniramine, and clemastine prolonged the action potential duration in guinea-pig isolated papillary muscles at 90% repolarization at I and $10\,\mu$m, respectively [68]. However, in contrast to the study above, others found that diphenhydramine had no effect on action potential duration in isolated papillary muscles [68] or QT interval in guinea-pigs [69].

Despite these studies, there has been relatively few data on the proarrhythmic risk of these first generation antihistamines on humans, with the exception of diphenhydramine, being the most frequently used antihistaminic drug. In one study on 126 patients (mean age 26 ± 11 years) [70] who had diphenhydramine suicidal overdose (in majority of cases the dose was >500 mg), the QTc duration was significantly longer compared with healthy subjects (453 ± 43 vs. 416 ± 35 ms, respectively, $P < 0.001$). The mean T-wave amplitude was significantly lower (0.20 ± 0.10 vs. 0.33 ± 0.15 mV, respectively, $P < 0.001$) but paradoxically, the dispersion of repolarization was significantly lower in diphenhydramine-overdose patients than in control subjects (42 ± 25 vs. 52 ± 21 ms, respectively; $P = 0.003$). None of the diphenhydramine-overdose patients experienced TdP. Thus, diphenhydramine overdose is associated with a significant but moderate QTc prolongation but none of the studied patients, including those who had apparent QTc prolongation, experienced TdP.

Thus, among the first generation antihistamines, their proarrhythmic risks remain unclear and contradictory with the evidence currently available.

Conclusion

Nonsedating antihistamines are widely prescribed for the treatment of allergic disorders. The overall evidence so far indicates that the potential to cause ventricular arrhythmias is not a class effect of nonsedating antihistamines and certain nonsedating antihistamines such as terfenadine and astemizole have potent proarrhythmic risk, whereas others have low risk of (e.g., azelastine, mizolastine) or are probably not associated with (e.g., loratadine, cetirizine, fexofenadine) QT prolongation, TdP or other ventricular arrhythmias. There is still a lack of information on the cardiac actions of some of the newer nonsedating antihistamines.

References

1 Craft TM. Torsades de pointes after astemizole overdose. *BMJ* 1986; 292: 6.
2 Simons FER, Kesselmann MS, Giddings NG, Pelech AN, Simons KJ. Astemizole-induced torsades de pointes. *Lancet* 1988; 45: 624.
3 Hoppu K, Tikanoja T, Tapanainen P, Remes M, Saarenpaa-Heikkila O, Kouvlainen K. Accidental astemizole overdose in young children. *Lancet* 1991; 338: 538.
4 Clark A, Love H. Astemizole-induced ventricular arrhythmia. an unexpected cause of convulsions. *Int J Cardiol* 1991; 33: 165–7.
5 Wiley JFII, Gelber ML, Henretig FM, Wiley CC, Sandhu F. Cardiotoxic effects of astemizole overdose in children. *J Pediatr* 1992; 120: 799–802.
6 Davies AJ, Harindra V, McEwan A, Ghose RR. Cardiotoxic effect with convulsion in terfenadine overdose. *BMJ* 1989; 298: 325.
7 McConnel TJ, Stanner AJ. Torsades de pointes complicating treatment with terfenadine. *BMJ* 1991; 302: 1469.
8 Broadhurst P, Nathan AV. Cardiac arrest in a young woman with the long QT syndrome and concomitant astemizole ingestion. *Br Heart J* 1993; 70: 469–70.
9 Venturini E, Borghi E, Maurini V, Vecce R, Carnicelli A. Prolongation of the QT interval and hyperkinetic ventricular arrhythmia probably induced by terfenadine use in liver cirrhosis patients. *Recenti Prog Med* 1992; 83: 21–2.
10 Monahan BP, Ferguson CL, Killeavy ES, Lloyd BK, Troy J, Cantilena LR. Torsades de pointes occuring in association with terfenadine use. *JAMA* 1990; 264: 2788–90.
11 Zechnich AD, Hedges JR, Eiselt-Proteau D, Haxby D. Possible interactions with terfenadine or astemizole. *West J Med* 1994; 160: 321–5.
12 Woosley RL, Chen Y, Freiman JP, Gilles RA. Mechanism of the cardiotoxic actions of terfenadine. *JAMA* 1993; 269: 1532–6.
13 Zhang M-Q. Chemistry underlying the cardiotoxicity of antihistamines. *Curr Med Chem* 1997; 4: 171–84.
14 Roy ML, Dumaine R, Brown AM. HERG, a primary human ventricular target of the nonsedating antihistamine terfenadine. *Circulation* 1996; 94: 817–23.
15 Surawicz B. Electrophysiologic substrate of torsades de pointes: dispersion of repolarization or early afterdepolarization. *J Am Coll Cardiol* 1989; 14: 172–84.
16 Ko CM, Ducic I, Fan J, Shuba YM, Morad M. Suppression of mammalian K+ channel family by ebastine. *Pharmacol Exp Ther* 1997; 281: 233–44.
17 Ducic I, Ko CM, Shuba Y, Morad M. Comparative effects of loratadine and terfenadine on cardiac K+ channels. *J Cardiovasc Pharmacol* 1997; 30: 42–54.
18 Suessbrich H, Waldegger S, Lang F, Busch AE. Blockade of HERG channels expressed in xenopus oocytes by the histamine receptor antagonists, terfenadine and astemizole. *FEBS* 1996; 385: 77–80.
19 Biton B, Maitre S, Godet D, Depoortere H, Arbilla S, O'Connor SE, Avenet P, Scatton B. Effect of the novel nonsedative histamine H1 receptor antagonist mizolastine on cardiac potassium and sodium currents. Allergy 1998: 53 (Abstract): 419.
20 Haria M, Fitton A, Peters DH. Loratidine. A reappraisal of its pharmacodynamic properties and therapeutic use in allergic disorders. *Drugs* 1994; 48: 617–38.

21 Taglialatela M, Pannaccione A, Castaldo P *et al*. The molecular basis for the lack of HERG K+ channels block-related cardiotoxicity by the H1 receptor blocker ceterizine as compared to other second-generation antihistamines. *Mol Pharmacol* 1998; 54: 113–21.

22 Lacerda AE, Roy M-L, Lewis EW, Rampe D. Interaction of the nonsedating antihistamine loratadine with a Kv1.5 type potassium channel cloned from human heart. *Mol Pharmacol* 1997; 52: 314–22.

23 Weissenburger J, Noyer M, Cheymol G, Jaillon P. electrophysiological effects of cetirizine, astemizole and d-sotalol in a canine model of long QT syndrome. *Clin Exp All* 1999; 29 (Suppl. 3): 190–6.

24 Woosley RL, Chen Y, Freiman JP, Gillis RA. Mechanism of the cardiotoxic actions of terfenadine. *JAMA* 1993; 269 (12): 1532–6.

25 Roy M-L, Dumaine R, Brown AM. HERG, a primary human ventricular target of the nonsedating antihistamine terfenadine. *Circulation* 1996; 94: 817–23.

26 Tillement JP. A low distribution Volume as a determinant of efficacy and safety for histamine (H1) antagonists. *Allergy* 1995; 50: 12–6.

27 Leeson GA, Chan KY, Knapp WC, Biedenbach SA, Wright GL, Okerholm RA. Metabolic disposition of terfenadine in laboratory animals. *Arzneimittelforschung* 1982; 32: 1173–8.

28 Michiels M, Van Peer A, Woestenborghs R, Heykants J. Pharmacokinetics and tissue distribution of astemizole in the dog. *Drug Dev Res* 1986; 8: 53–62.

29 Salata JJ, Jurkeiwicz NK, Wallace AA, Stupienski RF, Guinisso PJ, Lynch JJ. Cardiac electrophysiological actions of the histamines H1-receptor antagonists astemizole and terfenadine compared with chlopheniamine and pyrilamine. *Circ Res* 1995; 76: 110–9.

30 Honig PK, Wortham DC, Zamani K, Connor DP, Mulin JC, Cantilena LR. Terfenadine–ketoconazole interaction. *JAMA* 1993; 269: 1513–8.

31 Woosley RL. Cardiac actions of antihistamines. *Annu Rev Pharmacol Toxicol* 1996; 36: 233–52.

32 Hey JA, Del-Prado M, Kreutner W, Egan RW. Cardiotoxic and drug interaction profile of the second generation antihistamines ebastine and terfenadine in an experimental animal model of torsade de pointes. *Arzneim Forsch Drug Res* 1996; 46: 159–63.

33 Renwick AG. The metabolism of antihistamines and drug interactions: the role of cytochrome P450 enzymes. *Clin Exp All* 1999; 29 (Suppl. 3): 116–24.

34 Benton RE, Honig PK, Zamani K, Cantilena LR, Woosley RL. Grapefruit juice alters terfenadine pharmacokinetics, resulting in prolongation of repolarization on the electrocardiogram. *Clin Pharmacol Ther* 1996; 59 (4): 383–8.

35 Honig PK, Woosley RL, Zamani K, Conner DP, Cantilena LR Jr. Changes in the pharmacokinetics and electrocardiographic pharmacodynamics of terfenadine and concomitant administration of erythromycin. *Clin Pharmacol Ther* 1992; 52: 231–8.

36 Pratt CM, Ruberg S, Morganroth J *et al*. Dose–response relation between terfenadine (Seldane) and the QTc interval on the scalar electrocardiogram: distinguishing a drug effect from spontaneous variability. *Am Heart J* 1996; 131 (3): 472–80.

37 Moss AJ, Chaikin P, Garcia JD, Gillen M, Roberts DJ, Morganroth J. A review of the cardiac systemic side-effects of antihistamines: ebastine. *Clin Exp All* 1999; 29 (Suppl. 3): 200–5.

38 Malik M. Problems of heart rate correction in the assessment of drug induced QT interval prolongation. *J Cardiovasc Electrophysiol* 2001; 12: 411–20.

39 Lorber R, Danzig M, Brannan M. Loratadine (L) does not affect QTc interval nor produce torsades de pointes type arrhythmias. *Allergy* 1997; 37: 207.

40 Affrime MB, Lorber R, Danzig M, Cuss F, Brannan MD. Three months evaluation of electrocardiographic effects of loratidine in humans. *Allergy* 1993; 48 (Abstract); 1215.

41 Henz BM. The pharmacologic profile of desloratadine: a review. *Allergy* 2001; 56 (Suppl. 65): 7–13.

42 Kosoglou T, Salfi M, Lim JM, Batra VK, Cayen MN, Affrime MB. Evaluation of the pharmacokinetics and electrocardiographic pharmacodynamics of loratadine with concomitant administration of ketoconazole or cimetidine. *Br J Clin Pharmacol* 2000; 50: 581–589.

43 Abernethy DR, Barbey JT, Franc J, Brown KS, Feirrera I, Ford N, Salazar DE. Loratadine and terfenadine interaction with nefazodone, both antihistamines are associated with QTc prolongation. *Clin Pharmacol Ther* 2001; 69: 96–103.

44 Henz BM. The pharmacologic profile of desloratadine, a review. *Allergy* 2001; 56 (Suppl. 65): 7–13.

45 Kreutner W, Hey JA, Chiu P, Barnett A. Preclinical pharmacology of desloratadine, a selective and nonsedating histamine H1 receptor antagonist. Second communication, lack of central nervous system and cardiovascular effects. *Arzneimittelforschung* 2000; 50: 441–448.

46 Delauche-Cavallier MC, Chaufour S, Guerault E, Lacroux A, Murrieta M, Wajman A. QT interval monitoring during clinical studies with mizolastine, a new H1 antihistamine. *Clin Exp All* 1999; 29 (Suppl. 3): 206–11.

47 Sale ME, Barbey JT, Woosley RL, Edwards D, Yeh J, Thakker K, Chung M. The electrocardiographic effects of cetirizine in normal subjects. *Clin Pharmacol Ther* 1994; 54: 295–301.

48 Pratt C, Brown AM, Rampe D, Mason J, Russell T, Reynolds R, Ahlbrandt R. Cardiovascular safety of fexofenadine HCl. *Clin Exp All* 1999; 29 (3): 212–6.

49 Pratt CM, Mason J, Russell T, Reynolds R, Ahlbrandt R. Cardiovascular safety of fexofenadine HCL. *Am J Cardiol* 1999; 83: 1451–4.

50 Pinto YM, van Gelder IC, Heeringa M, Crijns HJ. QT lengthening and life-threatening arrhythmias associated with fexofenadine. *Lancet* 1999; 353 (9157): 980.

51 Anonymous. Severe cardiac arrhythmia on fexofenadine? *Prescrire Int* 2000; 9 (45): 212.

52 Craig-McFeely PM, Freemantle SL, Pearce GL, Shakir SA. QT lengthening and life-threatening arrhythmias associated with fexofenadine. *Br J General Pract* 2000; 50 (451): 148.

53 Kashyap AS, Kashyap S. Prolonged QTc time and ventricular arrhythmia with fexofenadine. *Am J Cardiol* 1999; 84 (10): 1278–9.

54 Giraud T. QT lengthening and arrhythmias associated with fexofenadine. *Lancet* 1999; 353 (9169): 2072–3.

55 DuBuske LM. Second-generation antihistamines. the risk of ventricular arrhythmias. *Clin Ther* 1999; 21 (2): 281–95.

56 Lang DG, Wang CM, Wenger TL. Terfenadine alters action potentials in isolated canine Purkinje fibers more than acrivastine. *J Cardiovasc Pharmacol* 1993; 22: 438–442.

57 Brannan MD, Reidenberg P, Radwanski E, Shneyer L, Lin C-C, Affrime MB. Evaluation of the pharmacokinetics and electrocardiographic parameters following 10 days of concomitant loratadine with ketoconazole. *J Clin Pharmacol* 1994; 34: 1016.

58 Brannan MD, Reidenberg P, Radwanski E, Shneyer L, Lin C-C, Cayen Mn Affrime MB. Loratadine administered concomitantly with erythromycin. pharmacokinetics and electrocardiographic evaluations. *Clin Pharmacol Ther* 1995; 58: 269–78.

59 Brannan MD, Affrime MB, Reidenberg P, Radwanski E, Lin C-C. Evaluation of the pharmacokinetics and electrocardiographic pharmacokinetics of loratadine with the concomitant administration of cimetidine. *Pharmacother* 1994; 14: 347.

60 Paserchia LA, Hewett J, Woosley RL. Effect of ketoconazole on QTc. *Clin Pharmacol Ther* 1994: 55 (Abstract): 146.

61 *Physician's Desk Reference*. Cetirizine prescribing information. Medical Economics Co., Montvale, NJ, 52nd edn 1998; 2234–6.

62 Lindquist M, Edwards IR. Risks of nonsedating antihistamines *Lancet* 1997; 349: 1322.

63 Cohen AT. Dangers of nonsedating antihistamines. *Lancet* 1997; 350: 69–70.

64 Himmel MH, Honig PK, Worobec AS. Dangers of nonsedating antihistamines. *Lancet* 1997; 350: 69–70.

65 de Abajo FJ, Rodriguez LA. Risk of ventricular arrhythmias associated with nonsedating antihistamine drugs. *Br J Clin Pharmacol* 1999; 47 (3): 307–13.

66 Passalacqua G, Bousquet J, Bachert C *et al*. The clinical safety of H1-receptor antagonists. *Allergy* 1996; 51: 666–75.

67 Wang WX, Ebert SN, Liu XK, Chen YW, Drici MD, Woosley RL. "Conventional" antihistamines slow cardiac repolarization in isolated perfused (Langendorff) feline hearts. *J Cardiovasc Pharmacol* 1998; 32 (1): 123–8.

68 Ki I, Inui A, Ito T. Effects of histamine H1 receptor antagonists on action potentials in guinea-pig isolated papillary muscles. *Arch Int Pharmacodyn Ther* 1996; 331 (1): 59–73.

69 Hey JA, Del Prado M, Cuss FM, Egan RW, Sherwood J, Lin CC, Kreutner W. Antihistamine activity, central nervous system and cardiovascular profiles of histamine H1 antagonists: comparative studies with loratadine, terfenadine and sedating antihistamines in guinea-pigs. *Clin Exp Allergy* 1995; 25 (10): 974–84.

70 Zareba W, Moss AJ, Rosero SZ, Hajj-Ali R, Konecki J, Andrews M. Electrocardiographic findings in patients with diphenhydramine overdose. *Am J Cardiol* 1997; 80 (9): 1168–73.

Risk of QT prolongation and torsades de pointes with psychotropic drugs

Background

The risk of sudden arrhythmic deaths associated with antipsychotics (e.g., thioridazine) has long been described but not fully appreciated [1,2]. In the 1960s, tricyclic antidepressants had also been recognized to have adverse cardiac effects and potentially fatal outcomes in overdose, and that the cause of these deaths was most often cardiovascular. It became clear subsequently that tricyclic antidepressants when taken either at or just above therapeutic levels prolonged intraventricular conduction and had a quinidine-like antiarrhythmic action [3], particularly on patients with pre-existing intraventricular conduction disease (bundle branch block, etc.) [4], as well as in patients with ischaemic heart disease [5].

While both thioridazine and tricyclic antidepressants had been regularly described to have "quinidine-like" action on the heart [6], the risk of proarrhythmia and sudden death with other antipsychotics was in dispute [7,8]. The assessment of the risk of antipsychotic-induced sudden death is made difficult by the fact that sudden deaths are rare events and psychotic patients have a substantially higher incidence of death, compared with the general population [9], due to natural as well as unnatural causes. Therefore, the causal relationship between some antipsychotics and arrhythmias or death is often difficult to establish. Nevertheless, autopsy evidence had already indicated that low-potency phenothiazines, especially thioridazine, were associated with sudden unexpected death in apparently healthy adults, although the mechanism behind these deaths was not then clear [10]. The discovery of the genetic mutations in patients with congenital long QT syndrome and the terfenadine story in the early 1990s have increased our understanding of the underlying mechanisms in drug-induced proarrhythmias and created a rational explanation for these early observations as well as increasing the awareness of proarrhythmia in psychotrophic treatment.

The concern about a relationship between QT prolongation, TdP and sudden death in antipsychotics has led to the withdrawal or restricted labeling of several antipsychotics worldwide. In 1996, a new atypical antipsychotic, sertindole, was not registered in the United States due to its effect on QT prolongation and association with 12 sudden unexplained deaths. Two years later, the Committee on Safety of Medicines (CSM) in the UK, which had previously approved the drug, found further evidence associating sertindole with malignant arrhythmia, and sertindole was voluntarily suspended from sale by the manufacturer. Sertindole is now being cautiously re-introduced into European Union countries. However, it carries a highly restrictive label to manage the risk of QT prolongation and TdP. In 2000, QT prolongation, TdP and sudden deaths had been reported with the use of thioridazine, and restricted labeling was introduced in both the United States and UK. Similarly, pimozide also received very restricted labeling for use in Tourette's syndrome.

Antipsychotics

Several new and some old antipsychotic drugs have now been implicated in QT prolongation, TdP and sudden death. The evidence for the association between fatal cardiac arrhythmias with antipsychotics is relatively new and mainly based on anecdotal case reports and case series published in scientific journals or notifications to regulatory authorities and pharmaceutical companies. Cardiac arrhythmias can occur at therapeutic doses or with overdose of the medication. However, the actual incidence of malignant arrhythmias is variable between different classes of antipsychotics. Furthermore, patients with schizophrenia are more likely to experience sudden death than the general population independent of drug treatment. It is therefore difficult to be sure that an antipsychotic is at fault. Sudden death could be the result of schizophrenic illness itself or illnesses related to the very high rate of smoking among such patients or a combination of the two [10,11]. None the less, increasing evidence has shown that certain antipsychotic carry a significant risk of proarrhythmia.

Butyrophenone antipsychotics (e.g., haloperidol, droperidol) have a reputation for safety and are free of many of the dangerous anticholinergic and cardiac side-effects of the lower potency neuroleptics. However, despite their efficacy and safety, there have been individual case reports and small series documenting QT prolongation, TdP and death related to therapy with oral or intravenous haloperidol in conventional doses to sedate agitated and delirious patients in the intensive care unit [12–16]. Cellular evidence has now confirmed that butyrophenones such as droperidol are potent I_{Kr} channel blockers even at therapeutic plasma concentrations (10–400 nmol/L) [17]. There have also been reports of haloperidol-, in some cases, droperidol-induced TdP in patients with conduction disturbance, bradycardia from sick sinus syndrome and hypokalaemia, all of which are known risk factors for TdP [15,18,19]. In a retrospective case-control study of 223 patients, two dozen well-documented cases of TdP were reported to be associated with the use of intravenous haloperidol in critically ill patients [20]. In this series, the risk of TdP associated with intravenous haloperidol treatment was estimated to be 3.6%, but rose to 11.1% if the dosage increased to >35 mg/day [20]. The risk of TdP with intravenous haloperidol increased if the QTc interval exceeded 500 ms with an odds ratio of 33 (95% CI: 6–195) compared with QTc interval ≤500 ms [20]. The risk of butyrophenone-induced QT prolongation and TdP, e.g., with droperidol, appears to increase when used intravenously in critically ill patients [18], when ECGs are frequently available before, during, and after an episode of drug-induced arrhythmia. On the other hand, the risk of a proarrhythmic effect with droperidol (or haloperidol) when prescribed orally to psychiatric patients is hard to assess and is currently unknown as there is almost never an ECG to document either the QT interval or TdP in psychiatric outpatient settings. On 31 March, 2001, droperidol (tablets, suspension and injection) was withdrawn voluntarily by its manufacturer in the UK following discussion with the Medicines Control Agency (MCA) following an extensive risk–benefit assessment.

Thioridazine, another antipsychotic, can cause marked QT prolongation, a decrease in T-wave amplitude, and a prominent U wave in approximately 50% of patients receiving 100–400 mg/day of the drug [21,22]. TdP can develop with thioridazine at therapeutic doses, and even with a low dose (50 mg daily) in the presence of hypokalaemia [23] [Figs 7.1 and 7.2]. At toxic

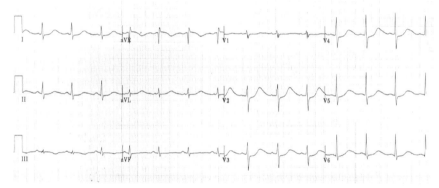

Fig. 7.1 The ECG of a middle-age woman who is otherwise healthy but suffered a ventricular fibrillation cardiac arrest while receiving 20 mg daily of thioridazine. This ECG was recorded immediately after the cardiac arrest (QTc = 619 ms).

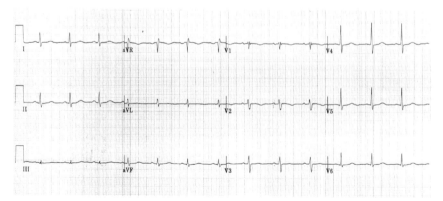

Fig. 7.2 The ECG of the same patient 3 days after the withdrawal of thioridazine (QTc = 399 ms).

levels, thioridazine can cause sinus bradycardia, atrioventicular block as well as marked QT prolongation, TdP, recurrent ventricular tachycardia and fibrillation [21,22]. Among thioridazine, chlorpromazine, pericyazine, trifluoperazine, haloperidol, prochlorperazine, fluphenazine or other neuroleptics, thioridazine was most potent in causing QT prolongation (QTc > 450 ms in 60% of patients), tachycardia, a widened QRS and ventricular arrhythmias [24], due to its blocking effect on the delayed rectifier I_{Kr} potassium channel and consequent abnormal repolarization [25]. Thioridazine exhibits a dose-dependent QT prolongation in healthy volunteers [26]. In July 2000, psychiatrists in the United States received a warning letter that thioridazine prolonged the QT interval and was associated with TdP and sudden death. On 11 December 2000, doctors in the UK also received a warning letter from the CSM on the cardiotoxcity and restricted use of thioridazine:

> "prescribing physicians are advised to perform baseline ECGs and serum electrolytes prior to initiation of thioridazine, and to repeat after each dose escalation and at 6-monthly intervals; the treatment should also be commenced with the lowest possible dose and to titrate slowly and be supervised by a consultant psychiatrist. The use of thioridazine should be restricted to second-line treatment of schizophrenia in adults, where other treatments have proved unsuitable, and that the balance of risks and benefits is unfavorable for its other previous indications."

Chlorpromazine is a phenothiazine that can prolong the QT interval but is more likely to do so if daily equivalent doses ≥2 g are used [27]. Chlorpromazine blocked I_{Kr} channels in isolated rat ventricular myocytes and induced early after-depolarizations in hypokalaemic isolated guinea-pig Purkinje fibers, which may explain its potential for QT prolongation and TdP [28,29]. However, so far there has only been one reported case of TdP (with T wave alternans, a risk marker of TdP) and cardiac arrest associated with its use [30,31].

Pimozide is a diphenylpiperidine neuroleptic agent with known cardiovascular side-effects including QT prolongation [32]. TdP has been described after acute poisoning [33]. Pimozide possesses electrophysiological effects similar to those of class III antiarrhythmic drugs. Experiments in native isolated ventricular myocytes demonstrated a concentration-dependent blockade of the I_{Kr} potassium current observed at recommended dosages of the drug [34]. Forty reports (16 fatal) of serious cardiac reactions (predominantly arrhythmias) with pimozide use had already been reported to the CSM between 1971 and 1995 [35] and restricted labeling has now been introduced for pimozide in the UK. Pimozide is strongly metabolized by cytochrome P450 CYP3A4 isoenzyme and special care should be taken to avoid potential pharmacokinetic interactions with the concomitant use of drugs that inhibit the cytochrome P450 CYP3A4 isoenzyme (e.g., clarithromycin, ketoconazole) that can lead to increase plasma levels and proarrhythmic risk of pimozide [36].

Atypical antipsychotics

Many new antipsychotics, the so-called atypical antipsychotics, have been introduced to the market recently because of their less potent extrapyramidal symptoms, notably clozapine analog atypical antipsychotics (clozapine, olanzapine and quetiapine) and serotonin-dopamine antagonist atypical antipsychotics (risperidone, sertindole and ziprasidone). However, these newer antipsychotics are not without adverse cardiac effects [37,38].

Although adverse cardiac events are rarely associated with risperidone therapy, prolongation of the QT interval has been reported to occur following two cases of presumed risperidone overdose and also in eight of 380 patients in a double-blind study reported by the manufacturer [39]. So far, there has been only a single case report of QT prolongation and fatal cardiac arrest associated with risperidone therapy but the underlying arrhythmia was unclear. No unequivocal case of risperidone-induced TdP has so far been reported.

Sertindole is a relatively new atypical antipsychotic for the treatment of schizophrenia, which was licensed in the UK in May 1996. Its safety and efficacy were assessed in three double-blind randomized studies in the United States, North America and Europe [40]. Slight QT prolongation was seen with sertindole in early clinical trials although TdP was not reported in these studies. However, 12 unexplained sudden deaths and 23 cases of syncope occurred among 1446 patients during the premarketing trials of sertindole [41]. A total of 27 deaths associated with its use had been reported to the Food and Drug Administration (FDA) by 1996. Although an independent review panel then did not find a causal relationship between sertindole and these deaths [42], the drug was not approved for marketing in the United States in 1996. Nevertheless, it was marketed in Europe. However, in the UK, the MCA/CSM were notified of 36 suspected adverse drug reactions with a fatal outcome by the end of November 1998 [43]. Not all of these reports were related to sudden cardiac death. In addition, 13 reports of serious but nonfatal cardiac arrhythmia were also reported in the UK during the same period. Because of the numbers of adverse drug events, fatal and nonfatal, reported since the marketing of sertindole in the UK, it was considered that the risks of sertindole therapy outweighed its benefits. The manufacturers of sertindole voluntarily suspended its marketing and use from 2 December 1998 in the UK pending further safety evaluations. It is now known that sertindole is a high affinity antagonist of the human cardiac I_{Kr} potassium channel and this blockade underlies, at least in part, the prolongation of the QT interval observed with this drug [44]. Sertindole showed a dose-dependent increase in the QTc interval that averaged 22 ms at usual therapeutic doses. However, sertindole is now being cautiously reintroduced in Europe. It is now evident that some of the QT prolongation is due to potentially antiarrhythmic activation of inward calcium currents. Many of the fatal cardiac events associated with use of sertindole occurred in patients who were receiving other drugs known to prolong the QT and cause TdP.

The adverse cardiac effects of other atypical antipsychotics such as olanzapine and clozapine are not yet clear. In an *in vivo* study of the isolated feline heart, haloperidol, risperidone, sertindole, clozapine and olanzapine prolonged the QT interval in a concentration-dependent manner [45]. Haloperidol and risperidone were significantly more potent than sertindole, clozapine and olanzapine. Haloperidol, risperidone, olanzapine and the newest serotonin-dopamine antagonist atypical antipsychotic, ziprasidone, are all I_{Kr} channel blockers [46].

Ziprasidone is known to prolong the QT interval [47]. The effect of ziprasidone and other antipsychotics on the QT interval is summarized in Figs 7.3 and 7.4. Phase II/III studies showed that short-term 4–6 weeks administration of ziprasidone (80–160 mg) prolonged the QTc interval by 5.9–9.7 ms (Bazett's formula) [48]. However, only 2/3095 (0.06%) ziprasidone-treated patients compared with 1/440 (0.23%) patients taking placebo developed QTc $\geq$ 500 ms, the threshold at which TdP is likely to occur. The incidence of QTc $\geq$ 500 ms with ziprasidone is less than 1/100th of that seen with sertindole which was reported to be 7.8%. Thus, ziprasidone has a small but unequivocal effect on repolarization that does not appear to be particularly dose dependent. Ziprasidone did not produce further QT prolongation when administered with the metabolic enzyme inhibitor ketoconazole. Although it has a 3A4 metabolic pathway, ziprasidone also has a major alde-

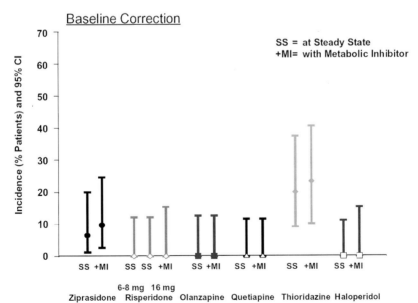

Fig. 7.3 Mean ΔQTc at steady state (SS) and in the presence of an appropriate P450 metabolic inhibitor (MI) (adapted from [48]).

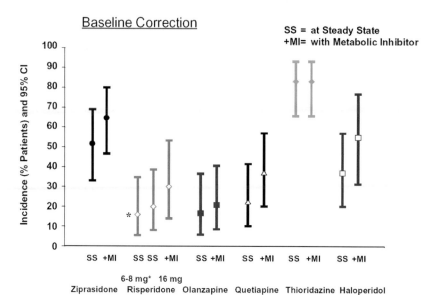

Fig. 7.4 Incidence of QTc ≥ 450 ms at steady state (SS) and with an appropriate P450 metabolic inhibitor (MI) (adapted from [48]).

hyde oxidase pathway, and this pathway is not known to be subject to either induction or inhibition. No report of TdP or excessive death compared with background has so far been documented with ziprasidone during the phase II/III studies [48]. In the study performed by Pfizer at the request of the FDA, ziprasidone prolonged the QT interval more than haloperidol, olanzapine, quetiapine, and risperidone but less than sertindole and thioridazine [48]. Thioridazine produced the most QT prolongation even though it was the only drug administered at less than half of its recommended maximal dose in this study. Although it is reassuring that ziprasidone was not associated with cardiac events during these premarketing trials, it does not guarantee that uncommon but life-threatening arrhythmias will not occur once the drug is in widespread use. Post-marketing surveillance is therefore required to monitor the risk of QT prolongation with ziprasidone.

Other less commonly used atypical antipsychotics including substituted benzamide atypical antipsychotics, amisulpride and sultopride, may also induce QT prolongation and TdP [49–51]. The duration of action potential of Purkinje fibers increased and early after-depolarizations noted with increased concentration of sultopride in cellular experiments [51].

The risk of drug-induced arrhythmias or sudden death is extremely difficult to estimate, mainly due to a lack of any controlled study. The only estimate available comes from a retrospective cohort study performed on Tennessee Medicaid enrollees that included 481 744 persons that were followed up for an average of 2.5 years from January 1988 to December 1993 (equivalent to 1 282 996 person-years of follow-up). In this study, 1487 subjects were confirmed to die from sudden cardiac deaths, equivalent to 11.6 per 10 000 person-years of observation [52]. The risk of sudden death for individuals receiving moderate-dose of antipsychotic drugs (> 100 mg thioridazine equivalents) was 2.39 times greater than for nonusers (95% CI = 1.77–3.22; $P < 0.001$). Among subjects with severe cardiovascular disease, the risk was even higher at 3.53-fold (95% CI = 1.66–7.51; $P < 0.001$) increased rate relative to comparable nonusers ($P < 0.001$), resulting in 367 additional deaths per 10 000 person-years of follow-up. Thus, patients that were prescribed moderate doses of antipsychotics had a significantly increased relative and absolute risk of sudden cardiac death, particularly for patients with cardiovascular disease. From these data, it was calculated that over a decade of exposure, there would be four extra deaths among 1000 apparently healthy young or middle-aged patients with schizophrenia who were treated with antipsychotic drugs [53]. This study, however, did not include the newer atypical agents such as risperidone.

Of note, similar to nonsedating antihistamines, many antipsychotics are metabolized by hepatic cytochrome P450 isoenzymes (Table 7.1). Thus, when prescribing these antipsychotics to patients, it is essential that coadministration of other drugs that inhibit the hepatic P450 isoenzymes are avoided to prevent toxicity of the vulnerable drugs. Other conditions that can inhibit the activity of hepatic cytochrome P450 isoenzyme include smoking, alcohol consumption and genetic polymorphism.

Tricyclic and related antidepressants

The most common cardiovascular adverse effects of tricyclic antidepressants (TCAs) are slowing of intraventricular conduction, manifested by prolonged PR, QRS on the ECG, and postural hypotension. In overdose, TCAs are fatal and the cause of these deaths is most often cardiovascular. Although it has been recognized previously that when taken either at or just above therapeutic levels, TCAs prolonged the intraventricular conduction and have a

Table 7.1 Antipsychotics and their hepatic metabolic pathway and corresponding metabolic enzyme inhibitor.

Drugs	Cytochrome P450 isoenzyme	Enzyme inhibitor
Haloperidol	CYP3A4, CYP2D6	Ketoconazole, paroxetine
Thioridazine	CYP2D6	Paroxetine
Quetiapine	CYP3A4	Ketoconazole
Olanzapine	CYP1A2	Fluvoxamine
Risperidone	CYP2D6	Paroxetine
Ziprasidone	CYP3A4	Ketoconazole

quinidine-like antiarrhythmic action, the increased use of TCAs, particularly in children, has raised some concern, especially with increasing reports of QT prolongation, TdP and unexpected deaths associated with their use.

An earlier survey on 153 cases of TCA poisoning (73% amitriptyline) showed that TCA poisoning caused QRS and QT prolongation in 42% of cases [54]. Interestingly, QRS but not QT duration was closely related to the severity of poisoning. In the presence of a hepatic cytochrome enzyme inhibitor, amitriptyline has also been reported to cause QT prolongation and TdP [55].

In children, desipramine use has been associated with sudden death (age 8–9) in the early 1990s [56,57]. Recently, two additional cases of sudden death in children treated with TCA were reported, one with desipramine and the other with imipramine [58]. Unfortunately, in most cases, the lack of information available did not allow the causal relationship between desipramine use and sudden death to be established. Nevertheless, Riddle and colleagues hypothesized that drug-induced long QT syndrome with desipramine use may be responsible [56] but the selective noradrenergic property of desipramine, which might increase cardiac sympathetic tone and predispose to ventricular tachyarrhythmias, is also possible as a cause of death [57], particularly in two cases where the children died shortly after exercise. Attempts at investigating the mechanism of sudden death with desipramine revealed mixed results. Johnson et al. did not observe any significant change on QT interval with desipramine and imipramine [59], whereas Leonard et al. noted that desipramine (and clomipramine) significantly prolonged the QT interval in children and adolescents [60]. The dosages and plasma concentrations of desipramine and clomipramine did not correlate with the changes in ECG parameters [60].

Despite the well-publicized reports above on the possible association of sudden death of children receiving desipramine, the systematic assessment of deaths of children receiving desipramine completed by the task force of the American Academy of Child and Adolescent Psychiatry did not support such an association [61]. A systematic literature search on Medline from 1967 to 1996 involving a total of 24 human studies (730 children and adolescents) given clomipramine, imipramine, amitriptyline, desipramine or nortriptyline [62] showed that imipramine had the greatest increase from baseline in the QTc interval, at 10% compared with clomipramine (5%), nortriptyline (4%) and desipramine (3%). However, desipramine had the highest incidence of significant QT prolongation (QTc > 440 ms) at 30%, compared with nortriptyline (17%), imipramine (16%), amitriptyline (11%) and clomipramine (11%). Recent cellular evidence confirmed that amitriptyline and imipramine exert their proarrhythmic effect by blocking the I_{Kr} channel, in a reversible manner [63,64]. The information on the arrhythmogenic mechanism of other antidepressants is currently lacking.

Desipramine and clomipramine are metabolized by at least three hepatic cytochromes; CYP3A4, CYP2C9 and CYP1A1/2, with CYP1A1/2 the major site of demethylation for tricyclic antidepressants [65]. Coadministration of drugs that can alter the levels of both parent drugs and metabolites will therefore affect the QTc interval [65]. Furthermore, there is a wide variation of both hydroxylation and demethylation of TCA, particularly in adults, influenced by age and race [65]. The multiplicity of cytochromes involved in demethylation and genetic polymorphism of CYP2DG and CYP1A1/2 give rise to "fast- or slow-metabolizers" and may explain the various adverse cardiac effect of TCAs [65,66]. More research is still needed to establish the long-term cardiac safety of TCAs, particularly in children. It is recommended that children and adolescents on TCAs receive an ECG at baseline and after each dose-increase [67]. Thus, the evidence shows that among the antidepressants, the tertiary tricyclic antidepressants (imipramine, amitriptyline and doxepin) appear to have a more general impact, while the secondary tricyclic antidepressants (nortriptyline, desipramine) may impact more on children and the elderly.

The proarrhythmic risk of other typical tricyclic antidepressants are less well described and the evidence has been mixed and less clear-cut. Cyclobenzaprine shares the same anticholinegic effects, tachycardia, and possibly dysrhythmic potential with tricyclic antidepressants. QT prolongation has been observed when cyclobenzaprine was coadministered with fluoxetine (which inhibits the hepatic cytochrome P450 CYP2D6, CYP3A4, CYP2C isoenzymes that metabolize cyclobenzaprine) [68]. In contrast, doxepin prolongs QT interval [69,70] and TdP has been reported with its use [71]. In patients with major depressive disorder, doxepin has been found to increase heart rate and significantly prolong QTc from 417 ± 36 to 439 ± 28 [72]. At the cellular level, doxepin (as well as thioridazine and chlorpromazine) induced early after-depolarizations under hypokalemic conditions in guinea-pig Purkinje fibers [73]. There has so far been no report of any TdP or arrhythmias associated with the use of lofepramine, trimipramine and amoxapine.

Newer tricyclic-related compounds such as mianserin, viloxazine, trazodone and maprotiline are thought to be safer in the proarrhythmic aspect but this is not exclusively the case. No report of QT prolongation, TdP or proarrhythmia has been reported in the literature on mianserin and viloxazine in contrast to trazodone and maprotiline. Trazodone, a second-generation antidepressant, has equal clinical efficacy as tricyclics. Although clinical trials have demonstrated a relatively safe arrhythmogenic profile, QT prolongation and polymorphic ventricular tachycardia have been observed with trasodone overdose [74] and with coadministration of trasodone and amiodarone [75]. Maprotiline is a tetracyclic anthracene-derivative antidepressant and is also used for the treatment of affective disorders. Although some studies have reported a low incidence of cardiovascular side-effects, others showed little difference between tetracyclic and tricyclic drugs. A few cases of QT prolongation and TdP have been reported with its use [76–79]. The arrhythmogenic mechanism of most tricyclic and related antidepressants is still not very clear, further study is required to determine whether they are all I_{Kr} blockers, similar to amitriptyline (i.e., a class effect).

In contrast to TCAs, selective serotonin reuptake inhibitors (SSRIs), including fluoxetine, dothiepin, and citalopram, are generally considered to cause less effect on cardiac impulse conduction and fewer cardiotoxic side-effects than TCAs. However, there are increasing numbers of case reports of dysrhythmias, such as atrial fibrillation, bradycardia and syncope associated with fluoxetine and another SSRI treatment and overdose. Although such reports have not been common, they do raise concerns.

So far the proarrhythmic effects of SSRIs as a group are rather mixed. For instance, dothiepin has no effect on QT interval at therapeutic dosage [80,81] and there has been no report of any TdP or arrhythmias associated with its use. Fluoxetine itself has not been known to prolong the QT interval in clinical or experimental studies [69,73] despite a reported case of QT prolongation [82] and a separate case report of TdP after poisoning with fluoxetine [83]. On the other hand, zimeldine, another SSRI, has been demonstrated to prolong the QT interval in rats [84] and in humans a case of QT prolongation and TdP has been reported [85]. Certain SSRIs such as fluoxetine and citalopram inhibit cardiac Na^+ and Ca^{2+} channels [86]. These direct cardiac electrophysiological effects are similar to those observed for tricyclic antidepressants, clomipramine and imipramine. It is unclear whether fluoxetine or other SSRIs are capable of blocking I_{Kr} or other potassium channels, which may explain their varying proarrhythmic potential.

Therapeutic doses of citalopram (up to 60 mg/day) have no long-term effect on cardiac conduction and repolarization in human patients [87], although it was found to have a small quinidine-like effect to decrease the amplitude of the R wave and reduce the later phase of depolarization [88]. In overdose, however, there has been controversy regarding the cardiac safety of citalopram.

While a number of reports state that citalopram is as safe in overdose as the other SSRIs [89,90], other researchers refute this conclusion [91,92]. Barbey and Roose [90] reported that in clinical trials, 15 patients overdosed on up to 2 g citalopram with no fatalities noted; the most common side-effects being nausea, somnolence, tachycardia, and sweating. However, Ostrom *et al.* [92] reported six cases of fatal overdoses in which citalopram was implicated as the cause of death. They suggested that a possible mechanism of death was cardiac arrhythmia [92]. After this initial report, the issue of withdrawal from the Swedish market was raised [93]. Grundemar *et al.* [94] reported five cases of citalopram overdose up to 5.2 g that had nonfatal outcomes but the patients developed significant ECG changes (prolonged QT intervals, tachycardia, and inferolateral repolarization disturbances), seizures, and rhabdomyolysis. There have also been a couple of anecdotal cases of QT prolongation and TdP with citalopram [95,96]. Furthermore, co-administration of other QT prolonging drugs with citalopram is common and associated with increased toxicity. There have been reports of mixed overdoses of citalopram/moclobemide, and citalopram/trimipramine that had fatal outcomes [97,98]. Thus, as a whole, citalopram is probably safe at therapeutic doses but has a slight increase in proarrhythmic risk when taken at overdose.

In a whole-cell patch clamp recording of heterologous HERG-mediated currents in transfected mammalian cells, citalopram blocks HERG with an IC [50] of 3.97 μm, which is slightly less potent than fluoxetine [49]. However, in isolated guinea pig ventricular cardiomyocytes, citalopram inhibited L-type calcium current (I_{Ca-L}). The effects of citalopram on both calcium current amplitude and the I_{Ca-L} "window" may help to explain citalopram's good cardiac safety profile, despite its propensity to block HERG at excessive dosages [99].

Chloral hypnotics

Chloral hydrate was previously frequently used as a hypnotic especially for children. Occasional arrhythmias including atrial fibrillation, aberrant conduction and premature ventricular contractions have been reported with chloral hydrate poisoning [100–102]. Rarely, overdose with chloral hydrate can lead to more serious dysrhythmia including QT prolongation and TdP [103,104]. Furthermore, there have also been some reports of unexplained death associated with oral ingestion of chloral hydrate in recommended dosage as well as in overdose [105–107]. Although the mechanism of deaths in these patients could not be established for certain, the toxic effect of chloral hydrate on ventricular repolarization could not be excluded as the cause of death. Further study is required to establish the pathomechanism behind the arrhythmogenic toxicity of chloral hydrate.

Lithium

The adverse proarrhythmic effect of lithium is controversial. There has so far been one case report of a patient with QT prolongation and T wave changes during lithium intoxication [108] and a patient with sinus bradycardia who developed TdP while receiving lithium and thioridazine [109]. In a recent study of QT interval abnormalities and psychotropic drug therapy in psychiatric patients [110], lithium therapy was not found to be associated with QT prolongation. However, lithium was the only drug among all the psychotropic drugs that was associated with nonspecific T wave abnormality (inverted, flattened or bifid T wave) [110]. Although lithium has been shown to decrease intracellular potassium level in sheep Purkinje fibers [111], its effect on the I_{Kr} channel is unknown and its role in acquired long QT syndrome is uncertain.

Abnormal ECG changes induced by psychotropic drugs mimicking Brugada syndrome

Recently, there have been some case reports of abnormal ECG changes akin to those observed on patients with Brugada's syndrome following the overdoses of antidepressants and neuroleptics, namely, phenothiazine, amitriptyline, desipramine, fluoxetine, and therapeutic doses of trifluoperazine

and loxapine, with tricyclic antidepressants being the most commonly implicated [112–114]. The ECGs in these patients showed right bundle branch block
and ST segment elevation on the precordial leads, similar to that seen in
patients with Brugada syndrome, following the ingestion of these drugs.
These changes, however, disappeared after the withdrawal of the drugs and
could not be reproduced with the subsequent flecainide tests on these patients.

In one study, on 98 consecutive patients, of intoxication with cyclic antidepressants (defined by a plasma concentration greater than $1\,\mu m/L$), a
Brugada electrocardiographic pattern was present in 15 of 98 cases (15.3%)
[115]. No patient had a personal or familial history of cardiac disease, and
none had ingested antiarrhythmic drugs. The prevalence of the Brugada
electrocardiographic pattern in patients with overdose of cyclic antidepressants exceeds the prevalence in the general population (0.05–0.1%). The
mortality rate was slightly higher at 6.7% among patients with the Brugada
electrocardiographic pattern compared with 2.4% among patients without it
but did not reach statistical significance [115]. The Brugada electrocardiographic pattern disappeared when plasma concentrations of cyclic antidepressants were less than $1\,\mu m/L$.

It has been suggested with evidence from cellular studies that, similar to
class Ic drugs, amitriptyline, phenothiazine and fluoxetine induce cardiac
sodium channel blockade and reduce I_{to} activation, both of which may
shorten the action potential durations and induce an intramyocardial electrical gradient that produces the typical ECG changes as described above
[112,115]. However, such ECG changes will probably only occur upon massive overdose of these drugs as in the case of these patients, which may
explain why the ECG changes could not be reproduced with the subsequent
flecainide challenge. Furthermore, it is also possible that these patients may
have subclinical dysfunctional sodium channels that were unmasked by
these drugs. Thus, it has been postulated that this could be another mechanism for drug-induced sudden death in patients on chronic treatment with
tricyclic antidepressants and neuroleptics. Nevertheless, further studies are
required to investigate this phenomenon further.

Conclusion

Among antipsychotic drugs, the low-potency phenothiazines, particularly
thioridazine, have been implicated most often in inducing QT prolongation,
TdP and sudden death. With a better understanding and awareness of
drug-induced proarrhythmia, the use of low-potency antipsychotic drugs
has became less common. They were replaced first by the high-potency
phenothiazines and butyrophenones and more recently by the atypical antipsychotics, many of which unfortunately appeared to possess proarrhythmic
risk as well. Among the atypical antipsychotics, the risk of QT prolongation
and TdP is variable. While sertindole, ziprasidone, risperidone, olanzapine,
quetiapine and clozapine have all been shown to prolong QT interval, only

sertindole has possibly been implicated in more than a few fatal and nonfatal arrhythmias, whereas risperidone has not been reported to induce TdP so far. Newer atypical antipsychotics such as ziprasidone require further evaluation and postmarketing surveillance to ascertain their cardiotoxicity although the premarketing trials so far suggest that TdP is not likely to be a serious problem with ziprasidone. Other neuroleptic agents such as pimozide (a diphenylpiperidine) have potent proarrhythmic risk and pimozide has now received restricted labeling for its use.

Among the antidepressants, the tertiary tricyclic antidepressants (imipramine, amitriptyline and doxepin) appear to have a more general impact on proarrhythmic effect, while the secondary tricyclic antidepressants (nortriptyline, desipramine) may have more impact on children and the elderly. In contrast to TCAs, selective serotonin reuptake inhibitors, including fluoxetine, dothiepin and citalopram, are generally considered to have less effect on cardiac conduction and cardiotoxic side-effects than TCAs.

Postmarketing surveillance after widespread use remains vital in the evaluation of any drug-induced proarrhythmia, especially on antipsychotics, as the data on high-risk patients such as frail, elderly patients or patients with preexisting cardiovascular disease in new drug application trials are very limited.

References

1 Kelly HG, Fay JE, Lavery SG. Thioridazine hydrochloride (Mellaril). its effects on the electrocardiogram and a report of two fatalities with electrocardiographic abnormalities. *Can Med Assoc J* 1963; 89: 546–54.

2 Fowler NO, McCall D, Chou TC, Holmes JC, Hanenson IB. Electrocardiographic changes and cardiac arrhythmias in patients receiving psychotropic drugs. *Am J Cardiol* 1976; 37: 223–30.

3 Glassman AH, Bigger JT Jr. Cardiovascular effects of therapeutic doses of tricyclic antidepressants: a review. *Arch General Psychiatry* 1981; 38: 815–20.

4 Roose SP, Glassman AH, Giardina EG, Walsh BT, Woodring S, Bigger JT. Tricyclic antidepressants in depressed patients with cardiac conduction disease. *Arch General Psychiatry* 1987; 44: 273–5.

5 Glassman AH, Roose SP, Bigger JT Jr. The safety of tricyclic antidepressants in cardiac patients: risk-benefit reconsidered. *JAMA* 1993; 269: 2673–5.

6 Lipscomb PA. Cardiovascular side-effects of phenothiazines and tricyclic antidepressants: a review. *Postgrad Med* 1980; 67: 189–96.

7 Leber P. Sudden death as a risk of neuroleptic treatment (a continuing controversy). *Psychopharmacol Bull* 1981; 17: 6–9.

8 American Psychiatric Association Task Force Report 27: Sudden Death in Psychiatric Patients: The Role of Neuroleptic Drugs. Washington, DC, APA, 1987.

9 Brown S. Excess mortality of schizophrenia, a meta-analysis. *Br J Psychiatry* 1997; 171: 502–8.

10 Mehtonen OP, Aranko K, Malkonen L, Vapaatalo H. A survey of sudden death associated with the use of antipsychotic or antidepressant drugs: 49 cases in Finland. *Acta Psychiatr Scand* 1991; 84: 58–64.

11 Dalack GW, Healy DJ, Meador-Woodruff JH. Nicotine dependence in schizophrenia. clinical phenomena and laboratory findings. *Am J Psychiatry* 1998; 155: 1490–501.

12 Kriwisky M, Perry GY, Tarchistsky D, Gutman Y, Kishon Y. Haloperidol-induced torsades de pointes. *Chest* 1990; 98 (2): 482–4.

13 Hunt N, Stern TA. The association between intravenous haloperidol and torsades de pointe. Three cases and a literature review. *Pyschosomatics* 1995; 36: 541–9.

14 Zee-Cheng CS, Mueller CE, Seifert CF, Gibbs HR. Haloperidol and torsades de pointes. *Ann Intern Med* 1985; 102: 418.

15 Fayer SA. Torsades de pointes ventricular tachyarrhythmia associated with haloperidol. *J Clin Psychopharmacol* 1986; 6: 375–6.

16 Metzger E, Friedman R. Prolongation of the corrected QT and torsades de pointes cardiac arrhythmia associated with intravenous haloperidol in the medically ill. *J Clin Psychopharmacol* 1993; 13 (2): 128–32.

17 Drolet B, Zhang S, Deschenes D *et al*. Droperidol lengthens cardiac repolarization due to block of the rapid component of the delayed rectifier potassium current. *J Cardiovasc Electrophysiol* 1999; 10 (12): 1597–604.

18 Lawrence KR, Nasraway SA. Conduction disturbances associated with administration of butyrophenone antipyshotics in the critically ill: a review of the literature. *Pharmacotherapy* 1997; 17 (3): 531–7.

19 Aunsholt NA. Prolonged QT interval and hypokalaemia caused by haloperidol. *Acta Psychiatr Scand* 1989; 79 (4): 411–2.

20 Sharma ND, Rosman HS, Padhi ID, Tisdale JE. Torsades de pointes associated with intravenous haloperidol in critically ill patients. *Am J Cardiol* 1998; 81: 238–40.

21 Kemper AJ, Dunlap R, Pietro DA. Thioridazine-induced torsades de pointes. Successful therapy with isoproterenol. *JAMA* 1983; 249: 2931–4.

22 Hulisz DT, Dasa SL, Black LD, Heiselman DE. Complete heart block and torsades de pointes associated with thioridazine poisoning. *Pharmacotherapy* 1994; 14: 239–45.

23 Denvir MA, Sood A, Dow R, Brady AJ, Rankin AC. Thioridazine, diarrhoea and torsades de pointes. *J R Soc Med* 1998; 91: 145–7.

24 Buckley NA, Whyte IM, Dawson AH. Cardiotoxicity more common in thioridazine overdose than with other neuroleptics. *J Toxicol Clin Toxicol* 1995; 33 (3): 199–204.

25 Drolet B, Vincent F, Rail J *et al*. Thioridazine lengthens repolarization of cardiac ventricular myocytes by blocking the delayed rectifier potassium current. *J Pharmacol Exp Ther* 1999; 288: 1261–8.

26 Hartigan-Go K, Bateman DN, Nyberg G, Martensson E, Thomas SH. Concentration-related pharmacodynamic effects of thioridazine and its metabolites in human. *Clin Pharmacol Ther* 1996; 60: 543–53.

27 Warner JP, Barnes TR, Henry JA. Electrocardiographic changes in patients receiving neuroleptic medication. *Acta Psychiatr Scand* 1996; 93 (4): 311–3.

28 Kon K, Krause E, Gogelein H. Inhibition of K^+ channels by chlorpromazine in rat ventricular myocaytes. *J Pharmacol Exp Ther* 1994; 271 (2): 632–7.

29 Studenik C, Lemmens-Gruber R, Heistracher P. Proarrhythmic effects of antidepressants and neuroleptic drugs on isolated, spontaneous beating guinea-pig Purkinje fibers. *Eur J Pharm Sci* 1999; 7 (2): 113–8.

30 Ochiai H, Kashiwagi M, Usui T, Oyama Y, Tokita Y, Ishikawa T. (Torsades de points with T wave alternans in a patient receiving moderate dose of chlorpromazine: report of a case). *Kokyu Junkan-Respiration Circulation* 1991; 38 (8): 819–22.

31 Cointe R, Dussarat GV, Mafart B, Bru P, Levy S. Arrhythmogenic effects of antidepressive agents demonstrated by programmed ventricular pacing. *Arch Mal Coeur Vaiss* 1989; 82 (3): 401–4.

32 Fulop G, Phillips RA, Shapiro AK, Gomes JA, Shapiro E, Nordlie JW. ECG changes during haloperidol and pimozide treatment of Tourette's disorder. *Am J Psychiatry* 1987; 144: 673–5.

33 Krahenbuhl S, Sauter B, Kupferschmidt H, Krause M, Wyss PA, Meier PJ. Case report. reversible QT prolongation with torsades de pointes in a patient with pimozide intoxication. *Am J Med Sci* 1995; 309 (6): 315–6.

34 Drolet B, Rousseau G, Daleau P, Cardinal R, Simard C, Turgeon J. Pimozide (Orap) prolongs cardiac repolarization by blocking the rapid component of the delayed rectifier potassium current in native cardiac myocytes. *J Cardiovasc Pharmacol Ther* 2001; 6 (3): 255–60.

35 CSM/MCA. Cardiac arrhythmias with pimozide (Orap). *Current Problems Pharmacovigilance* 1995; 21: 1.

36 Desta Z, Kerbusch T, Flockhart DA. Effect of clarithromycin on the pharmacokinetics and pharmacodynamics of pimozide in healthy poor and extensive metabolizers of cytochrome P450 2D6 (CYP2D6). *Clin Pharmacol Ther* 1999; 65 (1): 10–20.

37 Ravin DS, Levenson JW. Fatal cardiac event following initiation of risperidone therapy. *Ann Pharmacotherapy* 1997; 31: 867–70.

38 Rampe D, Murawsky MK, Grau J, Lewis EW. The antipsychotic agent sertindole is a high affinity antagonist of the human cardiac potassium channel HERG. *J Pharmacol Exp Ther* 1998; 286: 788–93.

39 Ravin DS, Levenson JW. Fatal cardiac event following initiation of risperidone therapy. *Ann Pharmacother* 1997; 31: 867–70.

40 Hale AS. A review of the safety and tolerability of sertindole. *Int Clin Psychopharmacol* 1998; 13 (3): S65–70.

41 Sertindole NDA 20–644. Rockville, Md, Food and Drug Administration, Psychopharmacological Drugs Advisory Committee, 1996.

42 Barnett AA. Safety concerns over antipsychotics drug, sertindole. *Lancet* 1996; 348: 256.

43 CSM/MCA. Suspension of availability of sertindole (serdolect). *Current Problems Pharmacovigilance* 1999; 25: 1.

44 Rampe D, Murawsky MK, Grau J, Lewis EW. The antipsychotic agent sertindole is a high affinity antagonist of the human cardiac potassium channel HERG. *J Pharmacol Exp Ther* 1998; 286 (2): 788–93.

45 Drici MD, Wang WX, Liu XK, Woosley RL, Flockhart DA. Prolongation of QT interval in isolated feline hearts by antipsychotic drugs. *J Clin Psychopharmacol* 1998; 18: 477–81.

46 Crumb WJ, Beasley C, Thornton A, Breier A. *Cardiac Ion Channel Blocking Profile of Olanzapine and Other Antipsychotics.* Presented at the 38th American College of Neuropsychopharmacology Annual Meeting; Acapulco, Mexico; December 12–16, 1999.

47 Shen WW. The metabolism of atypical antipsychotic drugs: an update. *Ann Clin Psychiatry* 1999; 11: 145–58.

48 FDA Psychopharmacological Drugs Advisory Committee. *Briefing Document for Zeldox (Ziprasidone Hcl).* New York: Pfizer Inc, 19 July 2000. www.fda.gov/ohrms/dockets/ac/oo/backgrd/361961a.pdf

49 Harry P. Acute poisoning by new psychotropic drugs. *Rev Prat* 1997; 47 (7): 731–5.

50 Tracqui A, Mutter-Schmidt C, Kintz P, Berton C, Mangin P. Amisulpride poisoning a report of two cases. *Hum Exp Toxicol* 1995; 14 (3): 294–8.

51 Lande G, Drouin E, Gauthier C, Chevallier JC, Godin JF, Chiffoleau A, Le Marec H. Arrhythmogenic effects of sultopride chlorhydrate: clinical and cellular electropysiological corrlation. *Ann Fr Anesth Reanim* 1992; 11 (6): 629–35.

52 Ray WA, Meredith S, Thapa PB, Meador KG, Hall K, Murray KT. Antipsychotics and the risk of sudden cardiac death. *Arch General Psychiatry* 2001; 58 (12): 1161–7.

53 Glassman AH, Bigger Jr. JT. Antipsychotic drugs: Prolonged QTc interval, torsade de pointes, sudden death. *Am J Psychiatry* 2001; 158: 1774–82.

54 Thorstrand C. Clinical features in poisoning by tricyclic antidepressants with special reference to the ECG. *Acta Med Scan* 1976; 199: 337–44.

55 Dorsey ST, Biblo LA. Prolonged QT interval and torsades de pointes caused by the combination of fluconazole and amitriptyline. *Am J Emerg Med* 2000; 18 (2): 227–9.

56 Riddle MA, Nelson JC, Kleinman CS, Rasmusson A, Leckman JF, King RA, Cohen DJ. Sudden death in children receiving Norpramin. a review of three reported cases and commentary. *J Am Acad Child Adolesc Psychiatry* 1991; 30: 104–8.

57 Riddle MA, Geller B, Ryan N. Another sudden death in a child treated with desipramine. *J Am Acad Child Adolesc Psychiatry* 1993; 32: 792–7.

58 Varley CK, McClellan J. Case study: two additional sudden death with tricyclic antidepressants. *J Am Acad Child Adolesc Psychiatry* 1997; 36: 390–4.

59 Johnson A, Giuffre RM, O'Malley K. ECG changes in pediatric patients on tricyclic antidepressants, desipramine, and imipramine. *Can J Psychiatry* 1996; 41: 102–6.

60 Leonard HL, Meyer MC, Swedo SE *et al.* Electrocardiographic changes during desipramine and clomipramine treatment in children and adolescents. *J Am Acad Child Adolesc Psychiatry* 1995; 35: 701–2.

61 Biederman J, Thisted RA, Greenhill L, Ryan N. Estimation of the association between desipramine and the risk of sudden death in 5- to 14-year old children. *J Clin Psychiatry* 1995; 56: 87–93.

62 Wilens TE, Biederman J, Baldessarini RJ *et al.* Cardiovascular effects of therapeutic doses of tricyclic antidepressants in children and adolescents. *J Am Acad Child Adolesc Psychiatry* 1995; 35: 1491–501.

63 Jo SH, Youm JB, Lee CO, Earm YE, Ho WK. Blockade of the HERG human cardiac K (+) channel by the antidepressant drug amitriptyline. *Br J Pharmacol* 2000; 129 (7): 1474–80.

64 Teschemacher AG, Seward EP, Hancox JC, Witchel HJ. Inhibition of the current heterologously expressed HERG potassium channels by imipramine and amitriptyline. *Br J Pharmacol* 1999; 128 (2): 479–85.

65 Oesterheld J. TCA cardiotoxicity: the latest. *J Am Acad Child Adolesc Psychiatry* 1996; 34: 1460–8.

66 Swanson JR, Jones GR, Krasselt W, Denmark LN, Ratti F. Death of two subjects due to imipramine and desipramine metabolite accumulation during chronic therapy: a review of the literature and possible mechanisms. *J Forensic Sci* 1997; 42: 335–9.

67 Alderton HR. Tricyclic medication in children and the QT interval: case report and discussion. *Can J Psychiatry* 1995; 40: 325–9.

68 Michalets EL, Smith LK, Van Tassel ED. Torsades de pointes resulting from the addition of droperidol to an existing cytochrome P450 drug interaction. *Ann Pharmacother* 1998; 32 (7–8): 761–5.

69 Baker B, Dorian P, Sandor P, Shapiro C, Schell C, Mitchell J, Irvine MJ. Electrocardiographic effects of fluoxetine and doxepin in patients with major depressive disorder. *J Clin Psychopharmacol* 1997; 17 (1): 15–21.

70 Giardina EG, Cooper TB, Suckow R, Saroff AL. Cardiovascular effects of doxepin in patients with ventricular arrhythmias. *Clin Pharmacol Ther* 1987; 42: 20–7.

71 Strasberg B, Coelho A, Welch W, Swiryn S, Bauernfeind R, Rosen K. Doxepin induced torsades de pointes. *Pacing Clin Electrophysiol* 1982; 5: 873–7.

72 Baker B, Dorian P, Sandor P, Shapiro C, Mitchell J, Irvine MJ. Electrocardiographic effects of fluoxetine and doxepin in patients with major depressive disorders. *J Clin Psychopharmacol* 1997; 17: 15–21.

73 Studenik C, Lemmens-Gruber R, Heistracher P. Proarrhythmic effects of antidepressants and neuroleptic drugs on isolated spontaneously beating guinea-pig Purkinje fibers. *Eur J Pharm Sci* 1999; 7 (2): 113–8.

74 Levenson JL. Prolonged QT interval after trasodone overdse. *Am J Psychiatry* 1999; 156 (6): 969–70.

75 Mazur A, Strasberg B, Kusniec J, Sclarovsky S. QT prolongation and polymorphic ventricular tachycardia associated with trasodone-amiodarone combination. *Int J Cardiol* 1995; 52 (1): 27–9.

76 Abinader EG. Q-T prolongation and torsades de pointes ventricular tachycardia produced by mapratiline. *Am J Cardiol* 1984; 53 (4): 654.

77 Herrmann HC, Kaplan LM, Bierer BE. Q-T prolongation and torsades de pointes ventricular tachycardia produced by the tetracyclic antidepressant agent maprotiline. *Am J Cardiol* 1983; 51 (5): 904–6.

78 Rialan A, Ricahrd M, Deutsch P, Ouattara B. Torsades de pointes in a patient under long-term maprotiline therapy. *Annales Cardiologie D'angeiologie* 1996; 45: 123–5.

79 Curtis RA, Giacona N, Burrows D, Bauman JL, Schaffer M. Fatal maprotiline intoxication. *Drug Intelligence Clin Pharmacy* 1984; 18: 716–20.

80 Claghorn JL, Schroeder J, Goldstein BJ, 2nd. Comparison of the electrocardiographic effect of dothiepin and amitriptyline. *J Clin Psychiatry* 1984; 45 (7): 291–3.

81 Claghorn JL, Schroeder J, Goldstein BJ. Comparison of the electrocardiographic effect of dothiepin and amitriptyline. *J Can Psychiatry* 1984; 45: 291.

82 Varriale P. Fluoxetine (Prozac) as a cause of QT prolongation. *Arch Intern Med* 2001; 161 (4): 612.

83 Lherm T, Lottin F, Larbi D, Bray M, Legall C, Caen D. Torsades de pointes after poisoning with fluoxetine alone. *Presse Med* 2000; 29 (6): 306–7.

84 Forsberg T, Lindbom LO. l Cardiovascular effects of Zimeldine and tricyclic antidepressants in conscious rats. *Acta Pharmacol Toxicol (Copenh)* 1983; 53 (3): 223–9.

85 Liljeqvist JA, Edvardsson N. Torsades de pointes tachycardias induced by overdosage of Zimeldine. *J Cardiovasc Pharmacol* 1989; 14 (4): 666–70.

86 Pacher P, Ungvari Z, Nanasi PP, Furst S, Kecskemeti V. Speculations on difference between tricyclic and selective serotonin reuptake inhibitor antidepressants on their cardiac effects. Is there any? *Curr Med Chem* 1999; 6 (6): 469–80.

87 Rasmussen SL, Overo KF, Tanghoj P. Cardiac safety of citalopram: prospective trials and retrospective analyzes. *J Clin Psychopharmacol* 1999; 19: 407–15.

88 Slavicek J, Paclt I, Hamplova J *et al.* Antidepressant drugs and heart electrical field. *Physiol Res* 1998; 47: 297–300.

89 Hale AS. Citalopram is safe [letter]. *Br Med J* 1998; 316: 1825.

90 Barbey JT, Roose SP. SSRI safety in overdose [Letter]. *J Clin Psychiatry* 1998; 59 (Suppl. 15): 42–8.

91 Power A. Drug treatment of depression: citalopram in overdose may result in serious morbidity and death. *Br Med J* 1998; 316: 307–8.

92 Ostrom M, Eriksson A, Thorson J *et al.* Fatal overdose with citalopram. *Lancet* 1996; 348: 339–40.

93 Sacsson G, Bergman U. Risks with citalopram in perspective [letter]. *Lancet* 1996; 348: 1033.

94 Grundemar L, Wohlfart B, Lagerstedt C *et al.* Symptoms and signs of severe citalopram overdose [letter]. *Lancet* 1997; 349: 1602.

95 Catalano G, Catalano MC, Epstein MA, Tsambiras PE. QTc Interval Prolongation Associated with Citalopram Overdose. *A Case Report Literature Rev Clin Neuropharmacol* 2001; 24 (3): 158–62.

96 Meuleman C, Jourdain P, Bellorini M *et al.* Citalopram and Torsades de Pointes. *A Case Report] Arch Mal Coeur Vaiss* 2001; 94 (9): 1021–4.

97 Neuvonen PJ, Pohjola-Sintonen S, Tacke U *et al.* Five fatal cases of serotonin syndrome after moclobemide-citalopram or moclobemide-clomipramine overdoses [letter]. *Lancet* 1993; 342: 1419.

98 Musshoff F, Schmidt P, Madea B. Fatality caused by a combined trimipramine-citalopram intoxication. *Forensic Sci International* 1999: 125–31.

99 Witchel HJ, Pabbathi VK, Hofmann G, Paul AA, Hancox JC. Inhibitory actions of the selective serotonin re-uptake inhibitor citalopram on HERG and ventricular l-type calcium currents. *FEBS Lett* 2002; 512 (1–3): 59–66.

100 DeGiovanni AJ. Reversal of chloral hydrate-associated cardiac arrhythmia by a beta-adrenergic blocking agent. *Anesthesiology* 1969; 31: 93.

101 Gustafson A, Svensson SE, Ugander L. Cardiac arrhythmias in chloral hydrate poisoning. *Acta Med Scand* 1977; 201 (3): 227–30.

102 Marshall AJ. Cardiac arrhythmias caused by chloral hydrate. *Br Med J* 1977; 2 (6093): 994.

103 Young JB, Vandermolen LA, Pratt CM. Torsade de pointes: an unusual manifestation of chloral hydrate poisoning. *Am Heart J* 1986; 112: 181–4.

104 Sing K, Erickson T, Amitai Y, Hryhorczuk D. Chloral hydrate toxicity from oral and intravenous administration. *J Toxicol Clin Toxicol* 1996; 34 (1): 101–6.

105 Jastak JT, Pallasch T. Death after chloral hydrate sedation: report of case. *J Am Dent Assoc* 1988; 116 (3): 345–8.

106 Houpt M. Death following oral sedation. *ASDC J Dent Child* 1988; 55 (2): 123–4.

107 Meyer E, Van Bocxlaer JF, Lambert WE, Piette M, De Leenheer AP. Determination of chloral hydrate and metabolites in a fatal intoxication. *J Anal Toxicol* 1995; 19 (2): 124–6.

108 Jacob AI, Hope RR. Prolongation of the Q-T interval in lithium toxicity. *J Electrocardiol* 1979; 12 (1): 117–9.

109 Liberatore MA, Robinson DS. Torsade de pointes: a mechanism for sudden death associated with neuroleptic drug therapy? *J Clin Psychopharmacol* 1984; 4 (3): 143–6.

110 Reilly JG, Ayis SA, Ferrier IN, Jones SJ, Thomas SHL. QTc-interval abnormalities and psychotropic drug therapy in psychiatric patients. *Lancet* 2000; 355: 1048–52.

111 Gow IF, Ellis D. Effect of lithium on the intracellular potassium concentration in sheep heart Purkinje fibres. *Exp Physiol* 1990; 75 (3): 427–30.

112 Rouleau F, Asfar P, Boulet S, Dube L, Dupuis JM, Alquier P, Victor J. Transient ST segment elevation in right precordial leads induced by psychotropic drugs: relationship to the Brugada syndrome. *J Cardiovasc Electrophysiol* 2001; 12: 61–5.

113 Tada H, Sticherling C, Oral H, Morady F. Brugada syndrome mimicked by tricyclic antidepressant overdose. *J Cardiovasc Electrophysiol* 2001; 12 (2): 275.

114 Babaliaros VC, Hurst JW. Tricyclic antidepressants and the Brugada syndrome: an example of Brugada waves appearing after the administration of desipramine. *Clin Cardiol* 2002; 25 (8): 395–8.

115 Goldgran-Toledano D, Sideris G, Kevorkian JP. Overdose of cyclic antidepressants and the Brugada syndrome. *N Engl J Med* 2002; 346 (20): 1591–2.

Risk of QT prolongation and torsades de pointes with antimicrobial and antimalarial drugs

Macrolide antibiotics

Macrolide antibiotics are widely used for a broad variety of infections including upper respiratory tract infection or pneumonia. Several recent anecdotal reports have identified that macrolide antibiotics (e.g., erythromycin) prolong QT interval (ranging from 560 ms to 700 ms) and induce TdP [1–5]. Furthermore, macrolide antibiotics also inhibit the hepatic cytochrome P450 3A4 isoenzyme and increase serum concentration of QT-prolonging drugs that are metabolized by the hepatic enzyme such as terfenadine. Most of the patients who developed TdP in these case reports were critically ill in the intensive care unit but others had ischaemic heart disease, congenital heart disease or congenital long QT syndrome. Some were otherwise well apart from the chest infection. Most cases of proarrhythmia on erythromycin have occurred with intravenous infusion. However, oral erythromycin prolonged QT interval by 13.8 ± 31 ms ($3.7\% \pm 7.9\%$) as a comparator drug in one study although the actual dosage and duration were unclear [6].

Erythromycin prolonged the action potential by inhibiting the delayed rectifier potassium current, I_{Kr} [7], preferentially in M cells compared to the epicardial or endocardial cells [8], and at higher concentrations (100–200 mg/L), inducing phase 2 and phase 3 early after-depolarizations which is the basis of its proarrhythmic tendency [7]. In one study on human HERG gene, all six macrolides examined (clarithromycin, roxithromycin, erythromycin, josamycin, erythromycylamine and oleandomycin) have been shown to inhibit I_{Kr} current in a concentration-dependent manner [9]. The IC_{50} values (the concentration that inhibits 50% of the delayed rectifier I_{Kr} potassium current) were clarithromycin, $32.9 \, \mu m$; roxithromycin, $36.5 \, \mu m$; erythromycin, $72.2 \, \mu m$; josamycin, $102.4 \, \mu m$; erythromycylamine, $273.9 \, \mu m$; and oleandomycin, $339.6 \, \mu m$ [9]. These findings imply that the blockade of HERG may be a common feature of macrolides.

In a prospective evaluation of critically ill patients, erythromycin significantly prolonged the QTc interval from a baseline of 524 ± 105 ms to 555 ± 134 m after slow infusion of the drug (mean rate 8.9 ± 3.5 mg/min) compared with controls who received cephalosporins and had no change in their QTc interval (from 423 ± 96 to 419 ± 96 ms after infusion) [10,11]. The extent of QT prolongation correlated strongly with the erythromycin infusion rate [12] and the QT-prolonging effect is rapid (approximately 15 min after the infusion, and the effect disappeared rapidly at 5 min after the infusion had been stopped) [13]. Therefore, intravenous erythromycin should always be administered as a slow infusion and ECG monitoring should accompany erythromycin therapy, particularly in critically ill patients. Erythromycin should never be rapidly administered intravenously as it can lead to TdP, circulatory arrest and death [14,15]. While QT prolongation with erythromycin is quite common, particularly in patients with heart disease, the incidence of TdP is rare despite the anecdotal cases reported [16].

Oral clarithromycin has also been reported to cause QT prolongation, TdP or ventricular tachycardia in several case reports [17–22]. Roxithromycin, a semisynthetic macrolide, has also been reported to prolong QT interval in a patient with ischaemic heart failure, itself a risk factor, with rapid normalization of the QT interval on withdrawal of the drug [22]. In contrast, azithromycin and dirithromycin do not cause any further increase in QT interval compared with placebo when given to healthy adults receiving terfenadine [23,24] but further evidence is needed before a conclusion can be made on whether the risk of QT prolongation and TdP by macrolides is a class effect.

Erythromycin has a synergistic effect in QT prolongation and may induce TdP when it is coadministered with other QT prolonging drugs such as quinidine [25], cisapride [26] and terfenadine [27]. Furthermore, all macrolides (except azithromycin) are hepatic cytochrome P450 3A4 inhibitors and should therefore not be given concomitantly with any QT-prolonging drugs that are metabolized by hepatic cytochrome P450 3A4 isoenzyme such as terfenadine and cisapride [26,28]. The risk of QT prolongation and TdP with other less commonly used macrolide antibiotics such as troleandomycin, josamycin, flurythromycin, ponsinomycin is less clear.

Azole antifungals

The azole antifungal agents including imidazoles (ketoconazoles and miconazoles) and trizoles (itraconazole and fluconazole) have been reported to cause QT prolongation, either when given alone or concomitantly with other drugs such as nonsedating antihistamines (primarily terfenadine and astemizole) and tricyclic antidepressant [29–33]. Ketoconazole prolongs the QT interval by blocking the I_{Kr} channel. Although the blocking effect on I_{Kr} channel by the azoles as a whole is less clear it is probably a class effect.

Similar to macrolide antibiotics, ketoconazole and itraconazole also inhibit the hepatic cytochrome P450 CYP3A4 isoenzyme. Therefore, coadministration of ketoconazole, fluconazole or itraconazole with another QT-prolonging drug that is metabolized by the cytochrome P450 CYP3A4 isoenzyme, such as terfenadine or amitriptyline, will result in a markedly prolonged QT interval and increase the risk of TdP [29–32].

Quinolone

A number of new fluroquinolones have recently been introduced. The older quinolones such as nalidixic acid have limited antimicrobial properties but the addition of fluoride to the original quinolone compounds yielded an essentially new class of drugs, the fluoroquinolones, which have a broader antimicrobial spectrum and improved pharmacokinetic properties. Quinolones can thus be classified into four generations according to the expanded antimicrobial spectrum of the more recently introduced fluoroquinolones and their clinical indications [34]. First-generation drugs (e.g., nalidixic acid, clinoxacin) achieve minimal serum levels. Second-generation quinolones (e.g., ciprofloxacin, ofloxacin, norfloxacin, enoxacin and lomefloxacin) have increased Gram-negative and systemic activity. Third-generation fluorinated quinolones, or fluoroquinolones (e.g., levofloxacin, sparfloxacin, moxifloxacin and gatifloxacin) have expanded activity against Gram-positive bacteria and atypical pathogens. Fourth-generation quinolone drugs (currently only trovafloxacin) add significant activity against anaerobes.

Despite a common mechanism of action, the quinolones can be differentiated within classes based on their antimicrobial spectrums of activity, pharmacokinetic properties and safety profiles, primarily as a result of their respective side-chain modifications [35]. For example, the 8-halogenated derivatives, including sparfloxacin and clinfloxacin, are most likely to cause photosensitivity, whereas the C7 substitute found in enoxacin and trovafloxacin is more likely to result in central nervous system reaction. Interaction with theophylline is more likely to be seen with agents containing modifications at positions 1, 7 and 8 with ciprofloxacin and enoxacin. As a class, the fluoroquinolones are generally well tolerated and safe. The incidence of adverse events varies significantly depending on the physicochemical structure of the specific agents [35]. The adverse effects associated with fluoroquinolones most commonly include gastrointestinal disturbances, central nervous system reactions and dermatological effects, and are generally mild in severity and reversible on cessation of treatment. Serious adverse events include photosensitivity associated with sparfloxacin, and severe liver toxicity associated with trovafloxacin that resulted in significant morbidity and mortality.

The risk of QT prolongation and potentially fatal ventricular arrhythmias associated with quinolones was highlighted following the withdrawal of grepafloxacin due to several cases of sudden death and TdP, which were not anticipated during initial drug development. However, the cardiotoxicity of quinolones as a group is not clear. While it has been suggested that the QT-prolonging effect of quinolones is a class effect [36], others have stated that the cardiotoxic potential of grepafloxacin and sparfloxacin is higher than those of other quinolones [37]. The data on the cardiotoxicity of quinolones in general are still scarce.

Grepafloxacin, a newly available fluoroquinolone, has been marketed in Europe since 1998 and in the US since 1997 until it was recently withdrawn in Europe due to its potential cardiotoxicity. During animal studies on both rabbit and dog models, grepafloxacin prolonged the QT interval more than ciprofloxacin after intravenous dosage of 10–30 mg/kg and ventricular tachycardia appeared at a dosage of 300 mg/kg [38]. In the phase I study on healthy volunteers, grepafloxacin was noted to mildly prolong the QT interval with a mean QTc prolongation of 10 ms [39]. However, since grepafloxacin was marketed, seven sudden deaths and several cases of TdP have been reported to be possibly associated with its use [40] and it was withdrawn voluntarily in Europe and the US in 1999 by its distributor. *In vitro* HERG assays demonstrated a 15% inhibition of I_{Kr} channel at a concentration of 10 μm and 87% inhibition at 300 μm.

Another fluoroquinolone, temafloxacin, introduced in the US in 1992, was also withdrawn from the market less than 4 months after its introduction, but primarily because of numerous reports (approximately 50 cases) of serious noncardiac adverse events, including three deaths [41]. The major noncardiac side-effects included hypoglycaemia in elderly patients as well as a constellation of multisystem organ involvement characterized by anaphylaxis, severe hemolytic anaemia, renal failure, abnormal liver function tests, hypoglycaemia and coagulopathy. The cardiotoxicity of temafloxacin is unclear.

Most data on the cardiac adverse effect of quinolones centred on a new fluoroquinolone, sparfloxacin, as it was the original fluoroquinolone described to be associated with proarrhythmia. Sparfloxacin was observed to prolong the QT interval in dogs during preclinical development of the drug [6]. In earlier clinical trials (Phase I/II), in a dose-escalating study of 200–800 mg loading dose, followed by doses of 100–400 mg/day, 10% of healthy volunteers showed a QTc interval >460 ms, signaling early in the drug's development the potential for life-threatening arrhythmias [6]. In a Phase III trial of therapy of community-acquired pneumonia, QTc prolongation was observed in 2.4% of cases receiving sparfloxacin. An integrated analysis of the safety data of sparfloxacin from six multicenter phase III trials, consisting of five double-blind, randomized, comparative trials of sparfloxacin (a 400-mg oral loading dose followed by 200 mg/day for 10 days) vs. standard comparative therapies (erythromycin, cefaclor, ofloxacin, clarithromycin, and ciprofloxacin) confirmed that the mean change in the QTc interval from baseline was significantly greater in sparfloxacin-treated patients (10 ms) than in patients given comparator drugs (3 ms), although no associated ventricular arrhythmias were detected [42]. In a separate small double-blind, randomized, placebo-controlled, crossover study of 15 healthy volunteers, sparfloxacin given at two different doses of 200 and 400 mg prolonged the QT interval to the same extent in 4% compared with placebo [43]. No significant reverse rate-dependence of QT interval was observed. However, another clinical study on 90 healthy male volunteers showed that increases in the placebo-adjusted mean change and mean maximum change in QT interval were dose related. The placebo-adjusted increases in the QTc interval on day 1 were 9, 16, and 28 ms after the subjects received 200 mg, 400 mg and 800 mg of sparfloxacin, respectively. The corresponding increases on day 4 steady state were 7, 12, and 26 ms, respectively. Soon after the introduction of sparfloxacin into the market in 1994, seven cases of cardiac-related adverse events were reported (three cases with ventricular tachycardia with two fatalities), all of which occurred in patients with underlying cardiac conditions (i.e., risk factors for QTc prolongation), during the European postmarketing surveillance of sparfloxacin [6]. In postmarketing studies there were 145 reports of QT-related events among 49 000 patients (FDA database).

These clinical results paralleled the *in vitro* ability of sparfloxacin to inhibit HERG channels. In an *in vitro* study on rabbit Purkinje fibers, Sparfloxacin prolonged the duration of action potential in a concentration-dependent manner. In contrast, ofloxacin and levofloxacin did not alter the action potential duration at various concentrations $(1–100\,\mu m)$ [44]. At low stimulation rates, the sparfloxacin-induced prolongation of the action potential was greater and early after-depolarizations occurred in a concentration-dependent manner. Thus, sparfloxacin exerts a pure class III electrophysiological effect whereas levofloxacin and ofloxacin apparently do not. Sparfloxacin was metabolized by the kidney and its clearance was reduced and plasma concentration raised in patients with moderate (CLcr 30–49 mL/min per $1.73\,m^2$) or severe (CLcr 10–29 mL/min per $1.73\,m^2$) renal insufficiency but increases did not appear to augment drug effects on the QT interval or enhance the risk for adverse events compared with patients with normal renal function [45]. It is yet uncertain whether sparfloxacin will cause an unacceptable incidence of spontaneous TdP, particularly in low-risk patients but an anecdotal case has been reported [46]. Sparfloxacin is not yet commercially available in the UK.

In a preclinical study on anesthetized rabbit models, no ventricular arrhythmia was seen with moxifloxacin at dosage up to 120 mg/kg whereas sparfloxacin induced ventricular tachycardia, including TdP in 50% (3/6 models) at similar dosage. Data from the worldwide phase III clinical trials showed that the degree of QTc prolongation measured at baseline and 2 h postdose on day 3–5 of 400 mg daily of oral moxifloxacin was slightly greater at 6 ± 26 ms $(n = 787)$ compared with 2 ± 23 ms with clarithromycin $(n = 136)$, with 0.4% of patients having QTc > 500 ms and 1.3% with ΔQTc > 60 ms whilst receiving moxifloxacin [47]. In a total of 6000 patients in Phase II–IV clinical trials, no cardiovascular morbidity or mortality attributable to prolongation of the QTc interval was noted. There are, as yet, no data concerning the possible clinical sequel of this effect in high-risk patients at risk of QT interval prolongation during the early phase of clinical trials [48]. In postmarketing surveillance, out of about 2 million spontaneous reports there was a single reported case of TdP in an elderly female patient with several risk factors for ventricular arrhythmia (hypokalaemia, CAD, digoxin and a pacemaker inserted for a sick sinus syndrome). More cases of likely TdP have now accumulated suggesting a risk of at least 1 per million prescriptions. Moxifloxacin is an I_{Kr} blocker and prolonged the

QT interval in a dose-dependent manner but did not exert reverse rate-dependency [49]. Moxifloxacin is about one-third as potent as sparfloxacin in blocking the I_{Kr} channel in mouse atrial cells. Moxifloxacin also blocked the I_{Ks} channel, and the action potential duration was prolonged by moxifloxacin at a concentration much higher than sparfloxacin (50 μm vs. 3 μm) [49]. Moxifloxacin was excreted by both renal and faecal routes. It has no effect on the hepatic cytochrome P450 enzyme but mild hepatic reactions can happen and are a class effect, usually presenting as mild transaminase level increases without clinical symptoms [36].

Gatifloxacin is an advanced-generation, 8-methoxy fluoroquinolone that is active against a broad spectrum of pathogens. Clinical studies have shown that gatifloxacin has limited potential to prolong the QT interval. In study on 55 volunteers using oral and intravenous doses of gatifloxacin ranging from 200 to 800 mg, the prolongation of the QTc interval was 2.9 $\pm$ 16.5 ms but no subject had a QTc interval >450 ms in this study [50]. No cardiovascular morbidity or mortality attributable to QTc prolongation has occurred with gatifloxacin treatment in over 4000 patients in Phase II/III clinical trials, including 118 patients concurrently receiving drugs known to prolong the QTc interval and 139 patients with uncorrected hypokalaemia (although ECG monitoring was not performed). In 15 752 patients with respiratory tract infection enrolled in Phase IV trails, including 4906 patients with underlying cardiovascular diseases, no arrhythmias were reported. Among 1 300 000 patients who received gatifloxacin, TdP was reported in two cases, both occurring in patients who received concomitant sotalol or fluconazole (known to prolong the QT interval), and in a patient with bradycardia, hypomagnesaemia and syncope of unknown cause [51]. Thus, the likelihood of QTc prolongation may increase with increasing concentrations of the drug and may potentially lead to TdP. Therefore, the recommended dose should not be exceeded. Pharmacokinetic studies between gatifloxacin and drugs that prolong the QT interval such as cisapride, erythromycin, antipsychotics, and tricyclic antidepressants have not been performed. Therefore, similar to other QT-prolonging drugs, gatifloxacin should be used with caution when given concurrently with these drugs, as well as in patients with ongoing proarrhythmic conditions, such as clinically significant bradycardia or acute myocardial ischemia. Gatifloxacin can be administered without dose modification in patients with hepatic impairment and does not interact with drugs metabolized by the cytochrome P450 enzyme family.

Levofloxacin has been used in more than 200 million prescriptions, with a good safety record. Although levofloxacin has been implicated in the causation of QT prolongation and TdP [52], it did not alter the action potential duration in an experimental study on rabbit Purkinje fibers [44]. The United States Food and Drug Administration's spontaneous reporting system documented 11 cases of TdP in 3 million treatments with levofloxacin [36]. Data reported to R.W. Johnson Pharmaceutical Research Institute and Ortho-McNeil Pharmaceuticals, the US marketer of levofloxacin, document TdP at a frequency of only 1 per million prescriptions, similar to the rate of TdP associated with ciprofloxacin [53]. In one report, 15 cases of QT-related ventricular arrhythmias or cardiac arrest per 10 million prescriptions have been documented, but without satisfactory details [54]. These reports generally involve patients who had concurrent medical conditions and the relationship to levofloxacin has not been established. These clinical data are in accord with animal experiments showing a lack of prolongation of the action potential in the rabbit Purkinje fiber model at levofloxacin concentrations of 1–100 μm (12–20 times the therapeutic serum concentration in man), compared with an effect caused by sparfloxacin that became evident at a concentration of 10 μm [44]. In the guinea-pig isolated right ventricular myocyte model, sparfloxacin, grepafloxacin, moxifloxacin and gatifloxacin at a concentration of 100 μm prolonged the action potential duration by 13–40%, whereas ciprofloxacin, trovafloxacin and levofloxacin prolonged the duration of the action potential by 0.6–3.3% [53].

In an observational study, the mean QTc prolongation was measured in 37 patients receiving levofloxacin treatment and averaged at 4.6 ms (range 47–92 ms). The risk factors for QTc prolongation in these patients were electrolyte disturbances in eight patients, and in six patients coadministration of trimethoprim–sulfamethoxazole, amiodarone, cisapride or fluoxetine. The frequency of the outliers defined as QTc > 60 ms from baseline or > 500 ms overall was 3% (one of 37) and 11% (four of 37), respectively, in this study. Of four patients with QTc > 500 ms, one patient, who took amiodarone concomitantly, developed TdP [54]. In a retrospective study of 23 patients who received a standard dose of 500 mg of levofloxacin daily and had ECGs during treatment, levofloxacin prolonged the QTc interval >60 ms in 9% of patients and absolute QTc interval prolongation greater than 500 ms was present in 17% of patients, one of whom developed TdP although this patient was also receiving amiodarone [52]. The manufacturer of levofloxacin is now required to conduct further electrophysiological studies to investigate the *in vitro* effect of levofloxacin and similar agents on the I_{Kr} channel and its dose-response to QT intervals in male and female normal volunteers over a broad age range, including subjects >65 years of age, including placebo and active control arms employing other antimicrobials including all the recommended doses.

Arrhythmogenic risk of quinolones—a class effect?

The cardiotoxicity of quinolones as a class remains controversial, partly because of a lack of data, especially on the newer quinolones that are yet to be marketed. The evidence so far suggested that QT prolongation does not seem to be a class effect of the fluoroquinolones and there are significant differences between the various members of this group of drugs in prolonging the QT interval or action potential duration, at least in animal models. For instance, as discussed earlier, Adamantidis demonstrated that sparfloxacin but not levofloxacin or ofloxacin prolonged the cardiac repolarization in rabbit Purkinje fibers [44]. Anderson and colleagues also showed that on a rabbit model, sparfloxacin had a far greater effect on the I_{kr} potassium channel than grepafloxacin and gatifloxacin, although all agents could cause ventricular arrhythmia [55]. Sparfloxacin had the greatest effect for blocking I_{Kr} channel with an IC_{50} of 0.23 μm compared with IC_{50} I_{Kr} (the concentration that inhibits 50% of the delayed rectifier potassium current) of 26.5 μm for gatifloxacin and IC_{50} of 27.2 for grepafloxacin [55]. In a comparative study using patch-clamp electrophysiology, it was shown that quinolones inhibited the human HERG potassium currents, but with widely differing potencies. Among the quinolones tested, sparfloxacin was the most potent compound, displaying an IC_{50} value of 18 μm, whereas ofloxacin was the least potent compound, with an IC_{50} value of 1420 μm. Other IC_{50} values were as follows: grepafloxacin, 50 μm; moxifloxacin, 129 μm; gatifloxacin, 130 μm; levofloxacin, 915 μm; and ciprofloxacin, 966 μm. Blockade of HERG channel by sparfloxacin displayed positive voltage dependence. In contrast to HERG, the KvLQT1/minK potassium channel was not a target for blockade by the fluoroquinolones. These results provided a mechanism for the QT prolongation observed clinically with administration of sparfloxacin and certain other fluoroquinolones, because free plasma levels of these drugs after therapeutic doses approximate those concentrations that inhibit HERG channel current. In the cases of levofloxacin, ciprofloxacin, and ofloxacin, inhibition of HERG occurs at concentrations much greater than those observed clinically. The data indicate that clinically relevant HERG channel inhibition is not a class effect of the fluoroquinolone antibacterials but is highly dependent upon specific substitutions within this series of compounds. Furthermore, there may be significant differences between quinolones as shown by the large difference in the arrhythmogenic doses, for instance, between grepafloxacin (10–30 mg/kg) and ciprofloxacin (300 mg/kg) [56].

In a recent study on an *in vivo* rabbit arrhythmia model, sparfloxacin, moxifloxacin, gatifloxacin, grepafloxacin have all been shown to block I_{Kr} channel with descending order. Similarly, sparfloxacin prolonged QT interval by 370 ± 30 ms, followed by moxifloxacin (270 ± 30 ms), grepafloxacin (280 ± 25 ms) and gatifloxacin (255 ± 23) [57]. In isolated canine Purkinje fibers, sparfloxacin, grepafloxacin, moxifloxacin and ciprofloxacin prolonged action potentials in a descending order [58]. The prolongation was inverse frequency-dependent with larger increases in action potential duration occurring when the stimulation frequency was reduced to 0.5 Hz [58].

The most comprehensive study was that by Hagiwara *et al.* [59]. They examined the effects of 10 fluoroquinolone antibacterial agents, namely, levofloxacin, sitafloxacin, trovafloxacin, ciprofloxacin, gemifloxacin, tosufloxacin, gatifloxacin, grepafloxacin, moxifloxacin and sparfloxacin, on action potentials recorded from guinea pig ventricular myocardium. Sparfloxacin prolonged action potential duration (APD) by about 8% at 10 μm and 41% at 100 μm. Gatifloxacin, grepafloxacin and moxifloxacin also prolonged APD at 100 μm by about 13%, 24% and 25%, respectively. In contrast, levofloxacin, sitafloxacin, trovafloxacin, ciprofloxacin, gemifloxacin and tosufloxacin had

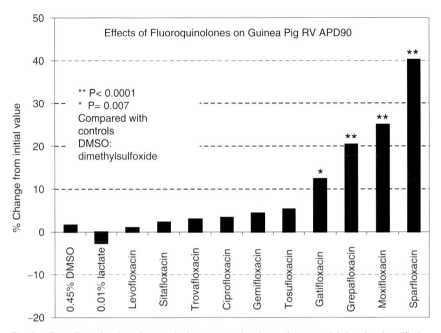

Fig. 8.1 The effect of various fluoroquinolones on prolonging action potential duration (modified from [59]).

little or no APD-prolonging effect at concentrations as high as $100\,\mu$m (Fig. 8.1). Thus, the evidence from all these studies suggests that there are significant differences in the potency to prolong QT interval among the fluoroquinolones and the risk of arrhythmia risk varies between drugs and with co-risk factors. Sporadic cases of TdP have been reported in association with most, but not all, fluoroquinolones. A blanket moratorium would therefore seem less appropriate than an objective assessment of risk. For instance, in a retrospective study in the United States between January 1st 1996 and May 2nd 2001, on the reported rate of quinolone-associated TdP, ciprofloxacin was associated with a significantly lower rate of TdP (0.3 cases/10 million prescriptions, 95% confidence interval [CI]: 0.0–1.1) than levofloxacin (5.4/10 million, 95% CI: 2.9–9.3, $P < 0.001$) or gatifloxacin (27/10 million, 95% CI 12–53, $P < 0.001$ for comparison with ciprofloxacin or levofloxacin) (Fig. 8.2) [60]. It is important to note that the reported rate used in this study is not synonymous with incidence rate and the numerators and denominators used in the rate calculations may be invalid. Nevertheless, information from spontaneous reports is generally useful as an early warning system for excess adverse events. As a whole, apart from sparfloxacin and possibly grepafloxacin, the fluoroquinolones that are currently on the market or soon to be launched are safe from the point of view of QT prolongation and TdP, with a frequency of this adverse event generally occurring at a reported rate of about 1 per million prescriptions. There is still a paucity of information and lack of objective data on the cardiac safety of other old and new quinolones including, norfloxacin, pefloxacin, fleroxacin, clinafloxacin, lomefloxacin, sitafloxacin, trovafloxacin, gemifloxacin, tosufloxacin and desquinolone. Figure 8.3 summarizes the effect of the few most commonly investigated quinolones on I_{Kr} blockade, action potential prolongation, QT prolongation and TdP.

Quinolones have a varying effect on the hepatic cytochrome P450 system. For instance, enoxacin and ciprofloxacin inhibit the hepatic cytochrome P450 enzyme system; others, such as ofloxacin and lomefloxacin have minimal effects on the system, whereas levofloxacin, gatifloxacin, and moxifloxacin have no effect at all on the system. Quinolones that inhibit hepatic cytochrome P450 enzyme should not be administered with other drugs that are metabolized via this enzymic system.

Antimalarials

Antimalarials deserve some attention as they are commonly prescribed worldwide. Quinine is the diastereomer of quinidine, and both drugs pro-

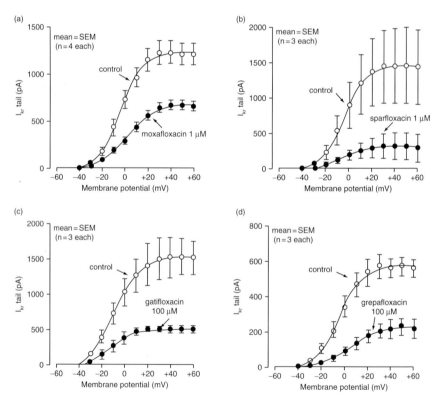

Fig. 8.2 (A) I_{Kr} blockade by quinolones (voltage clamp study) showing voltage dependence of I_{Kr} blockade with sparfloxacin being the most potent I_{Kr} blocker followed by grepafloxacin (equipotency as gatifloxacin) and moxifloxacin.

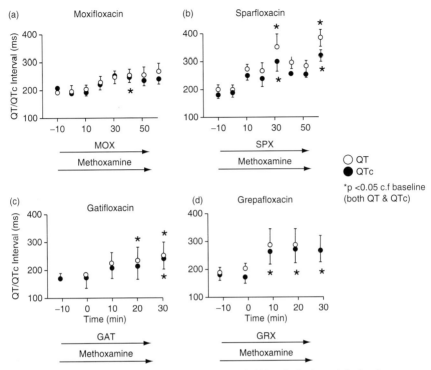

Fig. 8.2 (*cont'd*) **(B)** QT prolongation with quinolones (rabbit arrhythmia model) showing sparfloxacin is the most potent in prolonging the QT interval followed by grepafloxacin (equipotency as gatifloxacin) and moxifloxacin. (Modified from [60].)

	I_{kr} Blockade (Descending order)	↑ APD^*_{90} (Descending order)	↑ QT (ms)	TdP
Sparfloxacin			9–28 (200–800mg)	+ (rabbit/dog)
Grepafloxacin			10	+ (human)
Moxifloxacin			6±26	?
Gatifloxacin		?	2.9±16.5	?
Levofloxacin		–	>60ms (9% of pts)	+ (human)
Ciprofloxacin			?	+ (human)
Ofloxacin		–	?	?

*Canine or rabbit Purkinje fibers.

Fig. 8.3 The effect of various quinolones on I_{kr} blockade, action potential prolongation, QT prolongation and TdP.

duce prolongation of the QT interval. The threshold for the quinidine effect was lower than that for quinine but the change in QTc interval for a given change in free drug concentration was similar between the two drugs [61] although other workers have shown that QT prolongation was considerably greater in the quinidine compared to the quinine [62]. The change in QT interval is not predictive of the plasma concentration for quinine because the concentration within the therapeutic range produced only minor and unpredictable abnormalities.

The effect of QT prolongation (as well as QRS interval prolongation) with intravenous quinine infusion (given at 5 mg/kg over 5 min) was greatest between 1 and 4 min after completion of the quinine infusion [63]. The proarrhythmic risk of quinine is of particular concern in patients with acute renal failure especially after 3 days of therapy [64] and ECG monitoring may be advisable during quinine infusion in these patients.

The proarrhythmic risk of chloroquine is unclear despite two cases of TdP or ventricular fibrillation in the literature with chloroquine overdose [65,66]. Of note, both chloroquine and halofantrine caused significant inhibition of hepatic cytochrome CYP2D6 enzymic activity at therapeutic loading doses. Therefore, the combination of these drugs with other drugs known to prolong the QT interval should be avoided, especially those that are metabolized significantly by CYP2D6.

Halofantrine induced a PR and QT prolongation in adults with no pre-existing QT prolongation [67–69] and in children who received therapeutic dosage of halofantrine [70], as well as syncope, TdP and/or ventricular fibrillation in patients with congenital long QT syndrome [71,72]. Halofantrine induced a dose-related PR and QT prolongation and more than 60% of the effect occurred within three doses of halofantrine (24 mg/kg) [67]. Interestingly, significant QT prolongation (>25% or QTc ≥ 550 ms) was greater after halofantrine was used as a retreatment following mefloquine failure than as primary treatment. Although this might imply that mefloquine has a QT-prolonging tendency, another study did not support such a risk with mefloquine [68] and the potentiation of QT prolongation with halofantrine when used as a retreatment following mefloquine failure could be a result of mefloquine sensitization of halofantrine. Recent data confirmed that mefloquine does not prolong the QT interval or block the I_{Kr} channel but it does enhance the QT-prolonging effect of halofantrine by increasing the circulating concentration of halofantrine by 2–6-fold when given as a pretreatment before halofantrine [73]. Mefloquine does, however, block the slow delayed rectifier I_{Ks} potassium channel [74].

At standard dose of 24 mg/kg/day, halofantrine lengthened the QT interval duration from a mean QTc = 400 ms to 440 ms and the maximum QT interval with halofantrine treatment was observed at 12 h after administration [75]. The QTc interval significantly correlated with the plasma level of the parent drug halofantrine but not with the level of its plasma metabolite, N-desbutyl-halofantrine [76,77]. Like all QT-prolonging drugs, halofantrine is a potent inhibitor of the I_{Kr} channel with an IC_{50} value of 196.9 nm [78]. Blockade of I_{Kr} channel by halofantrine is predominantly due to high affinity binding to the open and inactivated channel states, with only a small contribution from lower affinity binding to closed channels. Halofantrine is very highly bound in whole blood (83% to serum proteins, 17% to erythrocyte), which may contribute partly to its potent cardiotoxicity [79]. In a study on open-chest anesthetized rabbits, halofantrine prolonged the QT interval in a dose-dependent manner and induced TdP in 4/6 of the animals studied and appeared to be more potent than terfenadine in its proarrhythmic toxicity [80]. Indeed, halofantrine is as potent as quinidine and class III antiarrhythmics in its ability to prolong repolarization [81].

Pentamidine

Since 1987, pentamidine has been reported to cause QT prolongation and TdP when given in intravenous form [82–93]. In addition, pentamidine can also induce tachycardia, hypotension, T wave inversion, ST segment depression [82,93] and U wave alternans [89]. Although it has been suggested that hypotension and tachycardia are probably part of the result of an autonomic vasodilatory effect or drug-induced histamine release rather than direct cardiac toxicity [94], the other electrocardiographic abnormalities such as T wave inversion and U wave alternans are very much the result of abnormal repolarization induced by pentamidine.

Stein et al. estimated that the cumulative incidence of QT prolongation (defined as QTc > 480 ms) was 27% after 7 days and 50% during 14 of 21 days of intravenous pentamidine therapy [95]. In their study, QT prolongation with pentamidine therapy always manifested within 2 weeks of the start of therapy although peak QT prolongation could occur as late as 5 days after the termination of the therapy. In another study, Eisenhauer et al. found that among the patients receiving intravenous pentamidine therapy with QT prolongation, the risk of TdP was 75% (3/4 patients) if QTc prolongation was >480 ms or 60% (3/5 patients) if ΔQTc was >80 ms [96]. The overall evidence suggested that the proarrhythmic risk of intravenous pentamidine appeared to be an idiosynchratic phenomenon rather than cumulative dose-related effects [96,97].

There is little information on the electrophysiological properties of pentamidine. However, it is known that pentamidine is structurally similar to procainamide [82] and it is therefore reasonable to postulate that pentamidine shares the same proarrhythmic properties of procainamide. Despite the cardiotoxicity of intravenous pentamidine [98], inhalator pentamidine is safe and did not prolong the QT interval, even when given at high dose (300 mg biweekly) for a prolonged period (>1 month) [99,100].

Pentavalent antimonial meglumine

Pentavalent antimony is used to treat leishmaniasis and has been noted to cause abnormal repolarization, including QT prolongation, flattened T waves, TdP and syncope [101–104]. Repolarization abnormalities were related to the total daily dose of antimony and duration of treatment. Repolarization abnormalities are common when pentavalent antimony is used at doses above 20 mg/kg/day for more than 15 days, and life-threatening arrhythmias may occur if very high doses are used [103], but QTc prolongation >500 ms has also been reported in 11% of patients receiving short-term, low-dose pentavalent antimony [104].

References

1 Gitler B, Berger LS, Buffa SD. Torsades de pointes induced by erythromycin. *Chest* 1994; 105: 368–72.

2 Guelon D, Bedock B, Chartier C, Harberer J. QT prolongation and recurrent torsades de pointes during erythromycin lactobionate infusion. *Am J Cardiol* 1986; 58: 666.

3 Katapadi K, Kostandy G, Katapadi M, Hussain KM, Schifter D. A review of erythromycin-induced malignant tachyarrhythmia – torsade de pointes. A case report. *Angiology* 1997; 48 (9): 821–6.

4 Brandriss MW, Richardson WS, Barold SS. Erythromycin-induced QT prolongation and polymorphic ventricular tachycardia (torsades de pointes): case report and review. *Clin Infect Dis* 1994; 18 (6): 995–8.

5 Rezkalla MA, Pochop C. Erythromycin induced Torsades de Pointes: case report and review of the literature. *S D J Med* 1994; 47 (5): 161–4.

6 Jaillon P, Morganroth J, Brumpt I, Talbot G and the Sparfloxacin Safety Group. Overview of electrocardiographic and cardiovascular safety data for sparfloxacin. *J Antimicrob Chemother* 1996; 37 (Suppl. A): 161–7.

7 Rubart M, Pressler ML, Pride HP, Zipes DP. Electrophysiological mechanisms in a canine model of erythromycin–associated long QT syndrome. *Circulation* 1993; 88: 1832–44.

8 Antzelevitch C, Sun ZQ, Zhang ZQ, Yan GX. Cellular and ionic mechanisms underlying erythromycin-induced long QT intervals and torsade de pointes. *J Am Coll Cardiol* 1996; 28 (7): 1836–48.

9 Volberg WA, Koci BJ, Su W, Lin J, Zhou J. Blockade of human cardiac potassium channel human ether-a-go-go-related gene (HERG) by macrolide antibiotics. *J Pharmacol Exp Ther* 2002; 302 (1): 320–7.

10 Tschida SJ, Guay DR, Straka RJ, Hoey LL, Johanning R, Vance-Bryan K. QTc-interval prolongation associated with slow intravenous erythromycin lactobionate infusions in critically ill patients: a prospective evaluation and review of the literature. *Pharmacotherapy* 1996; 16: 663–74.

11 Drici MD, Knollmann BC, Wang WX, Woosley RL. Cardiac action of erythromycin: influence of female sex. *JAMA* 1998; 280: 1774–6.

12 Haefeli WE, Schoenenberger RA, Weiss Ph, Ritz R. Possible risk for cardiac arrhythmia related to intravenous erythromycin. *Intensive Care Med* 1992; 18: 469–73.

13 Mishra A, Friedman HS, Sinha AK. The effects of erythromycin on the electrocardiogram. *Chest* 1999; 115 (4): 983–6.

14 Benoit A, Bodiou C, Villain E, Bavoux F, Checoury A, Badoual J. QT prolongation and circulatory arrest after an injection of erythromycin in a newborn infant. *Arch Fr Pediatr* 1991; 48 (1): 39–41.

15 Camilleri JF, Deharo JC, Panagides D *et al.* Jet intravenous injection of erythromycin lactobionate. A possible cause of the occurrence of crisis in torsade de pointe. *Ann Cardiol Angeiol (Paris)* 1989; 38 (10): 657–9.

16 Oberg KC, Bauman JL. QT interval prolongation and torsades de pointes due to erythromycin lactobionate. *Pharmacotherapy* 1995; 15: 687–92.

17 Lee KL, Jim MH, Tang SC, Tai YT. QT prolongation and torsades de pointes associated with clarithromycin. *Am J Med* 1998; 104: 395–6.

18 Kamochi H, Nii T, Eguchi K, Mori T, Yamamoto A, Shimoda K, Ibaraki K. Clarithromycin associated with torsades de pointes. *Jpn Circ J* 1999; 63 (5): 421–2.

19 Kundu S, Williams SR, Nordt SP, Clark RF. Clarithromycin-induced ventricular tachycardia. *Ann Emerg Med* 1997; 30: 542–4.

20 Sekkarie MA. Torsades de pointes in two chronic renal failure patients treated with cisapride and clarithromycin. *Am J Kid Dis* 1997; 30: 437–9.

21 Van Haarst AD, van't Klooster GA, van Gerven JM *et al.* The influence of cisapride and clarithromycin on QT intervals in healthy volunteers. *Clin Pharmacol Ther* 1998; 64: 542–6.

22 Woywodt A, Grommas U, Buth W, Rafflenbeul W. QT prolongation due to Roxifloxacin. *Postgrad Med J* 2000; 76: 651–4.

23 Harris S, Hilligoss DM, Colangelo PM, Eller M, Okerholm R. Azithromycin and terfenadine: lack of drug interaction. *Clin Pharmacol Ther* 1995; 58: 310–5.

24 Bachmann K, Sullivan TJ, Reese JH *et al.* A study of the interaction between dirithromycin and astemizole in healthy adults. *Am J Ther* 1997; 4 (2–3): 73–9.

25 Lin JC, Quasny HA. QT prolongation and development of torsades de pointes with the concomitant administration of oral erythromycin base and quinidine. *Pharmacotherapy* 1997; 17 (3): 626–30.

26 Michalets EL, Williams CR. Drug interactions with cisapride: clinical implications. *Clin Pharmacokinet* 2000; 39 (1): 49–75.

27 Honig PK, Wortham DC, Zamani K, Mullin JC, Conner DP, Cantilena LR. The effect of fluconazole on the steady-state pharmacokinetics and electrocardiographic pharmacodynamics of terfenadine in humans. *Clin Pharmacol Ther* 1993; 53: 630–6.

28 Fournier P, Pacouret G, Charbonnier B. A new cause of torsades de pointes: combination of terfenadine and troleandomycin. *Ann Cardiol Angeiol (Paris)* 1993; 42 (5): 249–52.

29 Zimmermann M, Duruz H, Guinand O, Broccard O, Levy P, Locatis D, Bloch A. Torsades de pointes after treatment with terfenadine and ketoconazole. *Eur Heart J* 1992; 13: 1002–3.

30 Pohjola-Sintonen S, Viitasalo M, Toivonen L, Neuvonen P. Itraconazole prevents terfenadine metabolism and increases risk of torsades de pointes ventricular tachycardia. *Eur J Clin Pharmacol* 1993; 45: 191–3.

31 Tsai WC, Tsai LM, Chen JH. Combined use of astemizole and ketoconazole resulting in torsades de pointes. *J for Med Assoc* 1997; 96: 144–6.

32 Dorsey ST, Biblo LA. Prolonged QT interval and torsades de pointes caused by the combination of fluconazole and amitriptyline. *Am J Emerg Med* 2000; 18 (2): 227–9.

33 Wassmann S, Nickenig G, Bohm M. Long QT syndrome and torsades de pointes in a patient receiving fluconazole. *Ann Intern Med* 1999; 131 (10): 797.

34 King DE, Malone R, Lilley SH. New classification and update on the quinolone antibiotics. *Am Fam Physician* 2000; 61 (9): 2741–8.

35 Bertino J Jr, Fish D. The safety profile of the fluoroquinolones. *Clin Ther* 2000; 22: 798–817.

36 Ball P, Mandell L, Niki Y, Tillotson G. Comparative tolerability of the newer fluoroquinolone antibacterials. *Drug Saf* 1999; 21 (5): 407–21.

37 Stahlmann R, Lode H. Toxicity of quinolones. *Drugs* 1999; 58 (Suppl. 2): 37–42.

38 Stahlmann R, Schwabe R. Safety profile of grepafloxacin compared with other fluoroquinolones. *J Antimicrob Chemother* 1997; 40 (Suppl. A): 83–92.

39 Summary of product characteristics. Raxar tablets. Glaxo Wellcome UK Limited.

40 Ball P. Quinolone-induced QT interval prolongation: a not-so-unexpected class effect. *J Antimicrob Chemother* 2000; 45: 557–9.

41 http://www.fda.gov/ohrms/dockets/ac/99/slides/3558s1/index.htm.

42 Lipsky BA, Dorr MB, Magner DJ, Talbot GH. Safety profile of sparfloxacin, a new fluoroquinolone antibiotic. *Clin Ther* 1999; 21 (1): 148–59.

43 Demolis JL, Charransol A, Funck-Brentano C, Jaillon P. Effects of a single oral dose of sparfloxacin on ventricular repolarization in healthy volunteers. *Br J Clin Pharmacol* 1996; 41: 499–503.

44 Adamantidis MM, Dumotier BM, Caron JF, Bordet R. Sparfloxacin but not levofloxacin or ofloxacin prolongs cardiac repolarization in rabbit Purkinje fibres. *Fundam Clin Pharmacol* 1998; 12: 70–6.

45 Dorr MB, Johnson RD, Jensen B, Magner D, Marbury T, Talbot GH. Pharmacokinetics of sparfloxacin in patients with renal impairment. *Clin Ther* 1999; 21 (7): 1202–15.

46 Dupont H, Timsit JF, Souweine B, Gachot B, Wolff M, Regnier B. Torsades de pointes probably related to sparfloxacin. *Eur J Clin Microbiol Infect Dis* 1996; 15 (4): 350–1.

47 http://www.fda.gov/cder/foi/label/1999/21085lbl.pdf.

48 Balfour JA, Lamb HM. Moxifloxacin. a review of its clinical potential in the management of community-acquired respiratory tract infections. *Drugs* 2000; 59 (1): 115–39.

49 http://www.fda.gov/ohrms/dockets/ac/99/transcpt/3558t2b.pdf.

50 http://www.fda.gov/cder/foi/label/1999/21062lbl.pdf.

51 Iannini PB, Circiumaru I. Gatifloxacin-induced QTc prolongation and ventricular tachycardia. *Pharmacotherapy* 2001; 21: 361–2.

52 Samaha FF. QTc interval prolongation and polymorphic ventricular tachycardia in association with levofloxacin. *Am J Med* 1999; 107: 528–9.

53 Kahn JB. Quinolone-induced QT interval prolongation: a not-so-unexpected class effect. *J Antimicrobial Chemotherapy* 2000; 46: 847–8.

54 Iannini P, Kramer H, Circiumaru I, Byazrova E, Doddmani S (2000). QTc prolongation associated with levofloxacin. In: *Program and Abstracts of the Fortieth Interscience Conference on Antimicrobial Agents and Chemotherapy, Toronto, Canada 2000 Abstract 822*. Washington, DC: American Society for Microbiology.

55 Anderson ME, Mazur A, Yang T, Roden DM. Potassium current antagonist properties and proarrhythmic consequences of quinolone antibiotics. *J Pharmacol Exp Ther* 2001; 296: 806–10.

56 Kang J, Wang L, Chen XL, Triggle DJ, Rampe D. Interactions of a Series of Fluoroquinolone Antibacterial Drugs with the Human Cardiac K (+) Channel HERG. *Mol Pharmacol* 2001; 59 (1): 122–6.

57 Anderson ME, Mazur A, Yang T, Roden DM. Potassium current antagonist properties and proarrhythmic consequences of quinolone antibiotics. *J Pharmacol Exp Ther* 2001; 296 (3): 806–10.

58 Patmore L, Fraser S, Mair D, Templeton A. Effects of sparfloxacin, grepafloxacin, moxifloxacin, and ciprofloxacin on cardiac action potential duration. *Eur J Pharmacol* 2000; 406 (3): 449–52.

59 Hagiwara T, Satoh S, Kasai Y, Takasuna K. A comparative study of the various fluor-oquinolones antibacterial agents on the cardiac action potential in guinea pig right ventricular myocardium. *Jpn J Pharmacol* 2001; 87: 231–4.

60 Frothingham R. Rates of torsades de pointes associated with ciprofloxacin, ofloxacin, levofloxacin, gatifloxacin, and moxifloxacin. *Pharmacotherapy* 2001; 21 (12): 1468–72.

61 Karbwang J, Davis TM, Looareesuwan S, Molunto P, Bunnag D, White NJ. A comparison of the pharmacokinetic and pharmacodynamic properties of quinine and quinidine in healthy Thai males. *Br J Clin Pharmacol* 1993; 35: 265–71.

62 White NJ, Looareesuwan S, Warrell DA. Quinine and quinidine: a comparison of ECG effects during the treatment of malaria. *J Cardiovasc Pharmacol* 1983; 5: 173–5.

63 White NJ, Chanthavanich P, Krishna S, Bunch C, Silamut K. Quinine disposition kinetics. *Br J Clin Pharmacol* 1983; 16 (4): 399–403.

64 Sukontason K, Karbwang J, Rimchala W, Tin T, Na-Bangchang K, Banmairuroi V, Bunnag D. Plasma quinine concentrations in falciparum malaria with acute renal failure. *Trp Med Int Health* 1996; 1: 236–42.

65 Collee GG, Samra GS, Hanson GC. Chloroquine poisoning: ventricular fibrillation following "trivial" overdose in a child. *Intensive Care Med* 1992; 18 (3): 170–1.

66 Demaziere J, Fourcade JM, Busseuil CT, Adeleine P, Meyer SM, Saissy JM. The hazards of chloroquine self prescription in west Africa. *J Toxicol Clin Toxicol* 1995; 33 (4): 369–70.

67 Nosten F, ter Kuile FO, Luxemburger C, Woodrow C, Kyle DE, Chongsuphajaisiddhi T, White NJ. Cardiac effects of antimalarial treatment with halofantrine. *Lancet* 1993; 341 (8852): 1054–6.

68 Laothavorn P, Karbwang J, Na Bangchang K, Bunnag D, Harinasuta T. Effect of meflo-quine on electrocardiographic changes in uncomplicated falciparum malaria patients. *South-east Asian J Trop Med Public Health* 1992; 23 (1): 51–4.

69 Gundersen SG, Rostrup M, von der Lippe E, Platou ES, Myrvang B, Edwards G. Halofantrine-associated ventricular fibrillation in a young woman with no predisposing QTc prolongation. *Scan J Infect Dis* 1997; 29 (2): 207–8.

70 Olivier C, Rizk C, Zhang D, Jacqz-Aigrain E. Long QTc interval complicating halofan-trine therapy in 2 children with plasmodium falciparum malaria. *Arch Pediatr* 1999; 6 (9): 966–70.

71 Monlun E, Leehardt A, Pillet O *et al.* Ventricular arrhythmia and halofantrine intake. Probable deleterious effect: Apropos three Cases. *Bull Soc Pathol Exot* 1993; 86 (5): 365–7.

72 Toivonen L, Viitasalo M, Siikamaki H, raatikka M, Pohjola-Sintonen S. Provocation of ventricular tachycardia by antimalarial drug halofantrine in congenital long QT syn-drome. *Clin Cardiol* 1994; 17 (7): 403–4.

73 Lightbown ID, Lambert JP, Edwards G, Coker SJ. Potentiation of halofantrine-induced QTc prolongation by mefloquine: correlation with blood concentrations of halofantrine. *Br J Pharmacol* 2001; 132 (1): 197–204.

74 Kang J, Chen XL, Wang L, Rampe D. Interactions of the antimalarial drug mefloquine with the human cardiac potassium channels KvLQT1/minK and HERG. *J Pharmacol Exp Ther* 2001; 299 (1): 290–6.

75 Matson PA, Luby SP, Redd SC, Rolka HR, Meriwether RA. Cardiac effects of standard-dose halofantrine therapy. *Am J Trop Med Hyg* 1996; 54 (3): 229–31.

76 Touze JE, Bernard J, Keundjian A, Imbert P, Viguier A, Chaudet H, Doury JC. Electro-cardiographic changes and halofantrine plasma level during acute falciparum malaria. *Am J Trop Med Hyg* 1996; 54 (3): 225–8.

77 Monlun E, Le Metayer P, Szwandt S, Neau D, Longy-Boursier M, Horton J, Le Bras M. Cardiac complications of halofantrine: a prospective study of 20 patients. *Trans R Soc Trop Med Hyg* 1995; 89 (4): 430–3.

78 Tie H, Walker BD, Singleton CB *et al.* Inhibition of HERG potassium channels by the antimalarial agent halofantrine. *Br J Pharmacol* 2000; 130: 1967–75.

79 Cenni B, Meyer J, Brandt R, Betschart B. The antimalarial drug halofantrine is bound mainly to low and high density lipoprotein in human serum. *Br J Clin Pharmacol* 1995; 39: 519–26.

80 Batey AJ, Coker SJ. Proarrhythmic potential of halofantrine, terfenadine and clofilium in a modified *in vivo* model of TdP. *Br J Pharmacol* 2002; 135 (4): 1003–12.

81 Wesche DL, Schuster BG, Wang WX, Woosley RL. Mechanism of cardiotoxicity of halofantrine. *Clin Pharmacol Ther* 2000; 67 (5): 521–9.

82 Wharton JM, Demopulos PA, Goldschlager N. Torsades de pointes during administration of pentamidine isethionate. *Am J Med* 1987; 83: 571–5.

83 Taylor AJ, Hull RW, Coyne PE, Woosley RL, Eliasson AH. Pentamidine-induced torsades de pointes: safe completion of therapy with inhaled pentamidine. *Clin Pharmacol Ther* 1991; 49: 698–700.

84 Stein KM, Haronian H, Mensah GA, Acosta A, Jacobs J, Kligfield P. Ventricular tachycardia and torsades de pointes complicating pentamidine therapy of *Pneumocystis carinii* pneumonia in the acquired immunodeficiency syndrome. *Am J Cardiol* 1990; 66: 888–9.

85 Lindsay J Jr, Smith MA, Light JA. Torsades de pointes associated with antimicrobial therapy pneumonia. *Chest* 1990; 98: 222–3.

86 Gonzalez A, Sager PT, Akil B, Rahimtoola SH, Bhandari AK. Pentamidine-induced torsades de pointes. *Am Heart J* 1991; 122: 1489–92.

87 Mitchell P, Dodek P, Lawson L, Kiess M, Russell J. Torsades de pointes during intravenous pentamidine isethionate therapy. *Can Med Assoc J* 1989; 140: 173–4.

88 Pujol M, Carratala J, Mauri J, Viladrich PF. Ventricular tachycardia due to pentamidine isethionate. *Am J Med* 1988; 84: 980.

89 Bibler MR, Chou TC, Toltzis RJ, Wade PA. Recurrent ventricular tachycardia due to pentamidine-induced cardiotoxicity. *Chest* 1988; 94: 1303–6.

90 Topol EJ, Lerman BB. Hypomagnesemic torsades de pointes. *Am J Cardiol* 1988; 52: 1367–8.

91 Cortess LM, Gasser RA Jr, Bjornson DC, Dacey MJ, Oster CN. Prolonged recurrence of pentamidine-induced torsades de pointes. *Ann Pharmacother* 1992; 26 (11): 1365–9.

92 Otsuka M, Kanumori H, Sasaki S *et al.* Torsades de pointes complicating pentamidine therapy of *Pneumocystis carinii* pneumonia in acute myelogenous leukemia. *Intern Med* 1997; 36 (10): 705–8.

93 Jha TK. Evaluation of diamidine compound (pentamidine isethionate) in the treatment of resistant cases of kala-azar occurring in North Bihar. *India Trans R Soc Trop Med Hyg* 1983; 77: 167–70.

94 Pearson RD, Hewlett EL. Pentamidine for the treatment of *Pneumocystis carinii* pneumonia and other protozoal diseases. *Ann Intern Med* 1985; 103: 782–6.

95 Stein KM, Fenton C, Lehany AM, Okin PM, Kligfield P. Incidence of QT interval prolongation during pentamidine therapy of *Pneumocystis carinii* pneumonia. *Am J Cardiol* 1991; 68: 1091–4.

96 Eisenhauer MD, Eliasson AH, Taylor AJ, Coyne PE Jr, Wortham DC. Incidence of cardiac arrhythmias during intravenous pentamidine therapy in HIV-infected patients. *Chest* 1994; 105: 389–94.

97 Girgis I, Gualberti J, Langan L, Malek S, Mustaciuolo V, Costantino T, McGinn TG. A prospective study of the effect of IV pentamidine therapy on ventricular arrhythmias and QTc prolongation in HIV-infected patients. *Chest* 1997; 112: 646–53.

98 Otsuka M, Kanamori H, Sasaki S *et al.* Torsades de pointes complicating pentamidine therapy of *Pneumocystis carinii* pneumonia in acute myelogenous leukemia. *Intern Med* 1997; 36 (10): 705–8.

99 Cardoso JS, Mota-Miranda A, Condo C, Moura B, Rocha-Goncalves F, Lecour H. Inhalatory pentamidine therapy and the duration of the QT interval in HIV-infected patients. *Int J Cardiol* 1997; 59 (3): 285–9.

100 Thalhammer C, Bogner JR, Lohmoller G. Chronic pentamidine aerosol prophylaxis does not induce QT prolongation. *Clin Invest* 1993; 71 (4): 319–22.

101 Ortega-Carnicer J, Alcazar R, De la Torre M, Benezet J. Pentavalent antimonial-induced torsade de pointes. *J Electrocardiol* 1997; 30 (2): 143–5.

102 Segura I, Garcia-Bolao I. Meglumine antimoniate, amiodarone and torsades de pointes: a case report. *Resuscitation* 1999; 42 (1): 65–8.

103 Chulay JD, Spencer HC, Mugambi M. Electrocardiographic changes during treatment of leishmaniasis with pentavalent antimony (sodium stibogluconate). *Am J Trop Med Hyg* 1985; 34 (4): 702–9.

104 Ribeiro AL, Drummond JB, Volpini AC, Andrade AC, Passos VM. Electrocardiographic changes during low-dose, short-term therapy of cutaneous leishmaniasis with the pentavalent antimonial meglumine. *Braz J Med Biol Res* 1999; 32 (3): 297–301.

Risk of QT prolongation and torsades de pointes with prokinetics and miscellaneous other drugs

Prokinetics

5HT$_4$ agonists

Cisapride is a gastrointestinal prokinetic agent used to treat gastroesophageal reflux disease, functional dyspepsia and delayed gastric emptying in adults. Its agonistic action at 5HT$_4$ receptors, thereby facilitating the cholinergic excitatory neurotransmission, has been suggested as the mechanism by which it enhances gastrointestinal motility. Cisapride has attracted much recent attention because of reports of QT prolongation, TdP, syncope and sudden death associated with its use [1–3]. An earlier report from the United States Food and Drug Administration (FDA) provided a first insight into the natural history of proarrhythmia associated with cisapride [4]. Between 1993 and 1996, the US FDA received reports of 34 cases of TdP and 23 cases of QT prolongation associated with cisapride use, of whom there were four deaths and 16 resuscitated cardiac arrests [4]. Many of the patients (56%) were also taking an imidazole compound or macrolide antibiotic, which could inhibit the P450 CYP3A4 isoenzyme that metabolizes cisapride and result in an increased serum level [5–7]. There were temporal associations between the onset of arrhythmia and increased serum level of cisapride, for instance during an increase in the dose, or the addition of an imidazole antifungal or macrolide antibiotic. In most patients, the arrhythmia stopped after the discontinuation of cisapride or the imidazole or macrolide antibiotic, or both. In some of the patients (9/15) tested for serum drug level from the FDA database, the serum cisapride levels were higher than the mean maximal levels found in clinical studies. QT prolongation and TdP recurred in two patients who were re-challenged with cisapride and one re-challenged with ketoconazole. Thus, the development of QT prolongation and TdP with cisapride appeared to be associated with conditions that inhibit its metabolism and the administration of high doses of cisapride. Several other risk factors that may have increased the risk of arrhythmia were also identified from this database: histories of coronary artery disease and arrhythmia (predominantly atrial fibrillation) (39%); renal insufficiency or renal failure (25%); electrolyte imbalance (19%) and; coadministration of QT prolonging drugs (12%) [4]. The risk for serious ventricular arrhythmia in an adult population has been estimated to be 1/120 000 patients but might be much higher because of underreporting [8].

Cisapride is a benzamine derivative and is structurally similar to procainamide [9]. At a molecular level, cisapride inhibited the I_{Kr} current in isolated guinea-pig ventricular myocytes in a concentration-dependent manner with an IC_{50} (concentration of half-maximum block) of 15 nmol/L (therapeutic levels, 50–200 nmol/L) [10]. In isolated rabbit cardiomyocytes, cisapride also blocked the I_{Kr} current in a concentration-dependent manner but at a lower $IC_{50} = 9$ nmol/L [11]. This explained the lengthening of cardiac repolarization observed in patients receiving clinical doses of cisapride. Cisapride also blocked the I_{Ks} channel but in a less potent manner than I_{Kr} blockade. *In vitro* study also showed that cisapride prolonged the duration of the monophasic action potential of anesthetized guinea-pig left ventricle and isolated rabbit Purkinje fibers. At very low frequency stimulation, cisapride could induce early after-depolarizations and triggered activity in Purkinje fibers. In a rabbit model of acquired long QT syndrome, the infusion of cisapride (0.3 μmol/kg/min for 10 min maximum) was associated with a significant QT prolongation of 43 ± 3.8 ms and the induction of TdP in 2/6 models. Thus, cisparide possesses the potent proarrhythmic property of a class III antiarrhythmic agent.

Cisapride has proved to be particularly proarrhythmic in infants when used in high dosage and several cases of QT prolongation and/or TdP have been reported [12–15]. Some of the infants and neonates were premature or extremely premature, and might have represented a high risk group due to their immature hepatic cytochrome P450 and renal secretion, which could increase the half-life and bioavailability of cisapride. Furthermore, cisapride is bound to albumin and hyperbilirubinaemia in premature neonates, which could cause displacement of cisapride. Several small prospective studies have been carried out to examine the causal relationship between cisapride use and its proarrhythmic risk. In two studies, children of various ages were prescribed cisapride at a dosage of 0.6–1.2 mg/kg/day. Both studies demonstrated that the incidence of prolonged QTc interval $\geq$450 ms with cisapride was 31% (11/35) and 13% (13/101), respectively [16,17]. In one of the studies, the mean ΔQTc was 15.5 ± 4.6 ms and ΔQTc >70 ms was seen in 3/35 patients [16]. Another study on seven small infants (age: 14–79 days; weight 1.2–4 kg; 6/7 premature) reported prolonged QT interval without arrhythmia while being on a large dose of cisapride (1–1.7 mg/kg/day) and the QT interval returned to normal within 48 h after the dose was reduced to a more modest dose of 0.8 mg/kg/day [18].

Despite these studies, several other prospective studies did not find an association between QT prolongation and cisapride use in dosage of 0.8 mg/kg/day (divided into four doses) in term healthy infants (age: 1.5–20 months) with QT interval measured 5 days after treatment [19] and premature infants with the QT interval measured 1 month after treatment [20]. A more recent study on full-term, small infants over 3 months of age (when hepatic cytochrome P450 CYP3A4 levels were still below adult levels), using cisapride at a dosage of 1 mg/kg/day only resulted in a slight nonsignificant increase in QT interval from 390 ± 18 ms to 400 ± 20 ms with no further change in QT interval even after 2 weeks of treatment. Only 2/100 infants in this study developed prolonged QTc interval >440 ms with no apparent risk factor [21].

Since cisapride was first marketed in 1988 in the UK, the Medicines Control Agency (MCA) has received reports of 60 serious cardiac adverse drug reactions from the UK, five of which were fatal. These included 24 reactions comprising ventricular arrhythmias, sudden unexplained death, cardiac arrest and QT prolongation [22]. Worldwide, there have been 386 reports of serious ventricular arrhythmias associated with cisapride therapy, 125 of which were fatal, and 50 reports of sudden unexplained death. In line with the earlier report from the FDA, the majority of these adverse reactions reported to the MCA occurred in patients who were taking contraindicated medication or who were suffering from underlying conditions known to increase the risk of ventricular arrhythmias. In the UK, cisapride has not been licensed for use in children and is specifically contraindicated in premature babies for up to 3 months after birth due to the risk of QT prolongation in this age group. Nevertheless, since marketing, 64 suspected adverse reactions in association with cisapride have been reported in the UK in children less than 13 years of age, including two cases of QT prolongation and two of sudden unexplained death [22]. A further 106 cardiovascular adverse events thought to be due to cisapride have also been received from other countries in children less than 13 years of age, including 30 cases of QT prolongation, four sudden unexplained deaths and six cases of ventricular fibrillation or tachycardia.

In the United States, while cisapride was being marketed from 1993 to 1999, the FDA received reports on a total of 341 individual patients who had serious adverse cardiac effects following the use of cisapride: 117 who developed QT prolongation; 107 TdP; 16 polymorphic ventricular tachycardia; 27 ventricular tachycardia; 18 ventricular fibrillation; 25 cardiac arrest; 16 serious (unspecified) arrhythmia; and 15 sudden death [23]. Eighty (23%) of the 341 patients died. Deaths were directly or indirectly associated with an arrhythmic event. As described earlier, factors that suggested an association with cisapride included a temporal relationship between use of cisapride and arrhythmia, the absence of identified risk factors and other explanations for arrhythmia in some patients, and cases of positive dechallenge and rechallenge. In most individuals, the arrhythmia occurred in the presence of risk factors (other drugs and/or medical conditions).

There were at least 30 drugs listed in the product information that could potentially interact with cisapride and the intake of cisapride with grapefruit juice may also increase its bioavailability (by inhibiting the gastrointestinal cytochrome P450 3A4 isoenzyme). In addition, special precautions are also needed in patients with renal or respiratory failure, significant heart disease, electrolyte imbalance or diabetes mellitus. As a result, the MCA suspended the product licences for cisapride in the UK in July 2000 as the risks and benefits balance was no longer considered favorable. Similarly, in the United States, the risk of fatal arrhythmia with cisapride was believed to outweigh the benefit for the approved indication, treatment of nocturnal heartburn, leading to the drug's discontinuation in the US.

New 5HT$_4$ agonists

New prokinetics that are currently under development include mosapride and tegaserod. Mosapride is a benzamide derivative, structurally related to cisapride, currently undergoing preclinical and clinical evaluation. Using isolated Langendoff-perfused rabbit hearts, mosapride did not prolong the duration of the monomorphic action potential or induce early after-depolarization and triggered activity in isolated rabbit Purkinje fibers. Mosapride blocked the I$_{Kr}$ current but at a markedly higher concentration than cisapride. Mosapride was approximately 1000-fold less potent than cisapride in blocking the I$_{Kr}$ current with an IC$_{50}$ = 4 μmol/L. One case of tiapride-induced TdP has been reported in the literature [24]. Zocapride is another 5HT$_4$-receptor agonist but in contrast to cisapride and mosapride, shortened the action potential duration in guinea-pig isolated papillary muscle [25].

Tegaserod did not prolong the QT interval at a concentration of between 0.5 and 10 μm, but the QT interval was significantly increased by 12 $\pm$ 4% if the concentration of tegaserod was increased to 50 μm (equivalent to 500–5000$\times$ the concentration typically found in human plasma after administration of recommended clinical dosages). In contrast, in the same models, cisapride significantly increased the QT interval by 22 $\pm$ 4% at a low concentration of 0.1 μm, and increased markedly to >70% when a concentration of 5–50 μm was used. Tegaserod metabolites had no effect on the QT interval [26]. Postmarketing surveillance will be required to monitor the safety of these new prokinetic agents.

Dopamine-receptor antagonist—domperidone

Domperidone is a prokinetic dopamine-receptor antagonist. As a result of the proarrhythmic risk of cisapride, domperidone has been felt to be a safer alternative to cisapride, due to its "apparent" favorable safety profile. However, QT prolongation, life-threatening ventricular tachyarrhythmias and cardiac arrest have been reported after the use of intravenous domperidone [27–34]. It has generally been assumed that these adverse events were related to the underlying electrolyte disturbance, e.g., hypokalemia, and not a drug effect. It is now known that similar to cisapride, domperidone is a potent I$_{Kr}$ blocker and prolongs cardiac repolarization at clinically relevant drug concentrations [35]. Therefore, domperidone should not be considered as a no-risk alternative to cisapride.

Ketanserin (5HT$_2$ serotonin antagonist)

Ketanserin is both a serotonin and weak α_1-receptor antagonist, it has been evaluated as a treatment for hypertension and peripheral vascular disease. At the experimental level, ketaserin has been found to markedly prolong the action potential duration in rabbit ventricular myocardium [36], canine ventricular muscle, and Purkinje fibers [37]. Ketanserin blocked the rapid component of the delayed rectifier I$_{Kr}$ potassium current in guinea-pig ventricular myocytes, with little or no effect on the inward rectifier I$_{K1}$ potassium current [38]. Ketanserin also blocked the transient outward I$_{To}$ potassium current in rat ventricular myocyte [39]. Together, they account for the prolongation of the action potential by ketanserin.

In humans, ketanserin has been reported to cause QT prolongation, ventricular arrhythmias and TdP [40–42]. In healthy subjects, 40 mg b.i.d. of ketanserin significantly prolonged the QTc interval by a mean 29 ± 7 ms compared with the controls [43]. In the early Prevention of Atherosclerotic Complications with Ketanserin Trial, some patients were withdrawn from the ketanserin group due to prolonged QTc interval > 500 ms and a fatal interaction between ketanserin and potassium-losing diuretics was noted that resulted in a number of deaths. In retrospect, this is not surprising, given the fact that hypokalaemia increased the risk of QT prolongation and TdP [44].

In a study by the Multicentre Ketanserin Research Group on patients with hypertension or coronary artery disease, ketanserin (given at 20 mg twice daily for 1 week followed by 3 weeks of 40 mg twice daily) significantly prolonged the QT interval from mean QTc interval of 400 ms to 418 ms although only 30% of patients had ΔQTc > 30 ms [45]. No patient had QTc > 500 ms in this study. Despite a significantly higher incidence of ventricular premature beats, bigeminy and nonsustained ventricular tachycardia in the ketanserin group compared with placebo group, there was no difference in the incidence of ventricular arrhythmias between both groups [45].

Another study on hypertensive patients showed that ketanserin had a potent QT-prolonging effect [46]. A single dose of 40 mg of ketanserin prolonged the QTc interval for at least 8 h, with a significant maximum QTc increase of 35 ms after 2 h. During chronic dosing of 20 and 40 mg, b.i.d., the QTc interval was further prolonged by 46 and 45 ms, respectively, worse than that seen on healthy subjects. The ΔQTc can increase to 80 ms in some patients given a high dose of ketanserin (mean dose 167 mg/day). QT prolongation with ketanserin was dependent on the body weight, dose of ketanserin corrected for body weight and dosage of the drug but not to the plasma level.

Miscellaneous

Probucol

Probucol is a hypocholesterolemic agent used primarily for the treatment of type II hyperlipidaemia. It was introduced in the US in the 1970s. Recently,

probucol has attracted some interest because of its known antioxidant properties, which may inhibit the oxidation of LDL cholesterol that plays an
important part in the formation of the atherogenic foam cells. Probucol has
been shown to produce QT prolongation and fatal arrhythmias in experimental animals [47]. During the earlier clinical experience with this drug,
despite its QT-prolonging effect in humans [48], there has been no association
between probucol and arrhythmias or other adverse cardiac events [49]. It has
been suggested that there might have been species differences in the pharmacokinetic and cardiotoxicity of probucol [50]. For instance, the occurrence
of QT prolongation and/or arrhythmias in the monkey seemed to have been
dependent on a concomitant high fat intake, which is known to facilitate
gastrointestinal absorption of probucol. In humans, there is normally a very
poor gastrointestinal absorption and bioavailability of probucol.

However, later clinical experience showed that probucol was capable of
causing ventricular arrhythmia, namely TdP, syncope as well as its effect on
the QT interval [51–53]. At a daily dosage of 500–750 mg, probucol prolonged
the QTc interval from 410 ms to 431 ms after a mean duration of 28.8 months of
treatment in patients with hypercholesterolemia [54]. Others also confirmed
that the ΔQTc with probucol is remarkably consistent at 22 ms [55,56]. However, there have been conflicting results on the correlation between serum
probucol levels and the degree of QT prolongation and no definite conclusion
can be made [56–58]. The risk factors for probucol-induced QT prolongation
are: female gender, prolonged baseline QT interval and low serum albumin
level. Marked lengthening of the QT interval is more likely to occur in patients
with ischemic heart disease or short baseline QT interval [54].

Tacrolimus

Tacrolimus, also known as FK506, is an immunosuppressant that has been
associated with QT prolongation and TdP in transplant patients [59,60]. In
guinea-pig, intravenous tacrolimus induced a sustained QT prolongation at
therapeutic serum concentration. In contrast to quinidine-induced QT prolongation that disappeared as plasma concentrations decreased, tacrolimus-
induced QT prolongation persisted despite a decline in the plasma drug
concentration [61].

Vasopressin

Intravenous vasopressin, used to treat bleeding oesophageal varices, can
induce QT prolongation and TdP. Some of these patients also had accompanying risk factors including electrolyte imbalance including (e.g., hypokalaemia and hypomagnesemia), coadministration of QT-prolonging drugs
(e.g., haloperidol, droperidol, etc.) [62–66].

Adenosine

Adenosine has been reported to induce QT prolongation and TdP. However,
in the majority of cases, the patients were at risk of developing TdP, these

included: patients with congenital long QT syndrome (adult and children); and patients with acquired long QT syndrome from intracranial hemorrhage or drug and atrial flutter [67–71].

In patients with congenital long QT syndrome, intravenous adenosine results in marked slowing of sinus and ventricular rate and leads to increased sympathetic discharge, which may induce bradycardia-induced TdP in this subgroup of patients. It is probable that both effects are the prerequisites for adenosine-induced TdP, since the addition of beta-blockers did not induce TdP in a case study when adenosine was given at a higher dose, despite the appearance of abnormal T waves [68]. However, nonpause-dependent non-sustained polymorphic ventricular tachycardia has been described in adults with structurally normal hearts, immediately after receiving 6 mg of intra-venous adenosine [72]. Thus, it has been suggested that adenosine may have increased the spatial or temporal heterogeneity of ventricular refractoriness as well (in the same way as it did on the atrium) and together with its effect on enhancing sympathetic tone, provided the condition for re-entrant arrhythmias. However, evidence on this is lacking and further study is needed to establish the proarrhythmic mechanism of intravenous adenosine.

Organophosphate poisoning
Organophosphate poisoning causes toxic myocarditis and myocardial necro-sis [73] and can cause QT prolongation and TdP as well as sinus tachycardia [74,75]. The incidence of repolarization abnormality with organophosphate poisoning is extremely common. In one series, 134/168 (79.7%) of patients with organophosphate poisoning had QT prolongation, ST segment and T wave abnormalities [76]. In this series, 56/168 (33.3%) of the patients had ventricular arrhythmias. Compared with patients without QT prolongation, patients with organophosphate poisoning and QT prolongation had a signifi-cantly higher rate of mortality (19.6% vs. 4.8%) and respiratory failure (56.7% vs. 20.6%) [77]. Thus, measurement of the QT interval after organophosphate poisoning carries prognostic significance.

Cocaine
Cocaine is a local anesthetic with a potent sympathetic stimulatory effect. It blocks the reuptake of catecholamines at the adrenergic nerve endings, in-hibits monoamine oxidases, desensitizes peripheral organs to the effect of exogenous catecholamines, and may exert a direct cardiotoxic effect. Cocaine has been implicated in the genesis of ventricular fibrillation, QT prolongation and TdP [78,79]. In patients with cocaine abuse and abnormal myocardial repolarization, the presence of myocardial ischaemia may further predispose to lethal ventricular arrhythmias and sudden death [80]. In the canine heart, cocaine increased both atrial and ventricular refractory periods and produced rate-dependent increases in atrial, atrioventricular, His–Purkinje and ven-tricular conduction intervals. Thus, unlike class III antiarrhythmics, cocaine produced a rate-dependent increase in the QT interval that was greatest at

high heart rates [81]. In dogs, cocaine significantly increased the QTc interval from 298 ± 7 ms to 339 ± 8 ms within 1 min of intravenous infusion of the drug [82]. Such effect, however, disappeared 10 min after cocaine administration.

Papaverine

Papaverine, a potent coronary vasodilator, is commonly used to measure coronary blood flow velocity and coronary flow reserve using a coronary Doppler catheter. Intracoronary papaverine can result in marked prolongation of the QT interval and TdP [83–86]. In one study, polymorphous ventricular tachycardia was reported to occur in 1.3% of patients (5 of 391) who received intracoronary papaverine. The arrhythmia was significantly more common in women (4.4%, 4/91) than in men (0.3%, 1/301) and lasted less than 1 min in all cases in this study, converting spontaneously in four and requiring electrical cardioversion in one [87]. At a dosage of 6–12 mg, intracoronary papaverine significantly increased the corrected QTc interval on the electrocardiogram (430 ± 30 to 490 ± 70 ms) [88].

Intracoronary heparin

There has been no formal documentation of QT prolongation with intravenous or intracoronary heparin injection. Intracoronary heparin injection commonly produces abnormal repolarization with reversible deep T wave inversion. However, the authors have observed anecdotal cases of patients undergoing percutaneous coronary angioplasty who were given prophylactic intravenous coronary heparin injection and subsequently developed transient QT prolongation and TdP (Fig. 9.1). Further investigation is necessary to examine the potential hazard of proarrhythmia against the perceived benefit of intracoronary heparin injection.

Cesium

A rare case of cesium-induced TdP has been reported [89].

Other QT-prolonging drugs that have been withdrawn

Early reports of TdP associated with cardiac drugs incriminated not only antiarrhythmics, but antianginal agents such as bepridil and prenylamine, both of which have been well documented to cause TdP [90,91]. These antianginal agents have now been withdrawn from the market in most regulatory jurisdictions. Terodiline, an antispasmodic agent used to treat urinary incontinence, was withdrawn in the UK following 69 reported cases of serious arrhythythmias. Fourteen of these patients had sudden death and the remaining 55 patients had nonfatal arrhythmias including 37 patients with ventricular tachyarrhythmia, of which 24 were due to TdP. It is now clear that the proarrhythmic effect of terodiline is a consequence of the blockade of I_{Kr} current, which occurs in a concentration-dependent manner.

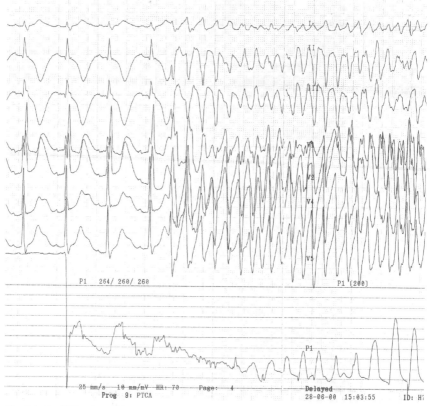

Fig. 9.1 The ECG of a patient undergoing percutaneous coronary angioplasty who developed QT prolongation and deep T wave inversion leading to self-terminating TdP after intracoronary heparin injection.

Bepridil

Early reports of TdP associated with cardiac drugs incriminated not only antiarrhythmics, but antianginal agents such as bepridil and prenylamine, both of which have been well documented to cause TdP [90, 91]. These antianginal agents have now been withdrawn from the market in most regulatory jurisdictions.

Bepridil is a unique calcium antagonist and initially developed as an antianginal agent but it has multiple electrophysiologic actions through class Ib, III, and IV mechanisms. It decreases calcium influx through potential-dependent and receptor-operated sarcolemmic calcium channels and acts intracellularly as a calmodulin antagonist and calcium sensitizer. Bepridil also shows a lidocaine-like fast kinetic block of inward sodium current. Finally, bepridil's blocks the outward potassium currents and inhibits the sodium–calcium exchange which increases the action potential duration and ventricular refractoriness. The final property forms the basis for a class III antiarrhythmic mechanism but also its proarrhythmic potential [92].

A major safety concern with bepridil is the occurrence of TdP associated with QT interval prolongation, especially in the context of hypokalemia with concomitant diuretic therapy [93]. In one study on patients with chronic stable angina, the mean QTc interval was significantly prolonged from 400 ms at baseline to approximately 450 ms at the end of 8 weeks of bepridil therapy [94]. Another study showed that bepridil prolonged the QTc interval by lesser extent at 5.6% [95].

Data from the US clinical trials of bepridil in 840 angina patients, bepridil (median dose, 300 mg/day) lengthened the rate-corrected QT interval in most patients. The mean increase was 7.7%. TdP occurred in 7 patients, an incidence of approximately 1%, all of whom were associated with low serum potassium level, or the use of a potassium-wasting diuretic [96]. Postmarketing surveillance data in France developed from 1981 to 1989 have revealed 108 validated episodes of torsades de pointes in patients treated with bepridil [97].

The effects of bepridil therapy on QTc intervals appeared to plateau after 14 days of treatment but in an individual whose initial QTc prolongation at day 14 was <40 ms, further QTc prolongation may still occur later. The degree of QT prolongation with bepridil is inversely proportional to the baseline QTc interval and heart rate [98]. Beta-blocker appeared to counteract and reduce the increase in QT interval, QT dispersion and TDR induced by bepridil [99].

Bepridil blocked both HERG and KvLQT1-IsK channels [100]. In rabbit Langendorff-perfused hearts, bepridil causes regionally different lengthening of APD in ventricular muscle leading to an increase in temporal dispersion of repolarization, which may be inducive for re-entrant arrhythmias when accompanied by slow conduction at toxic doses [101].

Mibefradil

Similarly, Mibefradil has also been reported to cause QT prolongation and torsades de pointes [102]. Bepridil and Mibefradil (as well as verapamil) blocked the HERG channel in a concentration-dependent manner, whereas nitrendipine and diltiazem have negligible effects. Similarly, KvLQT1/IsK is inhibited by bepridil and mibefradil, while being insensitive to nitrendipine, diltiazem, or verapamil. Thus, These results demonstrate that the cardiac delayed rectifier $K+$ current are sensitive targets to certain calcium channel blockers which may help in explaining the deleterious proarrhythmic effects associated with bepridil and mibefradil [103].

Prenylamine

Another antianginal agent, prenylamine, has also been implicated in inducing QT prolongation and life-threatening TdP [104–107]. The QT prolongation manifested after one week of daily 180 mg prenylamine treatment. The prolongation persisted as long as therapy was continued and returned to normal within 2 weeks of withdrawal of treatment [108]. Similar to the treatment for other drug-induced long QT syndrome and TdP, the TdP induced by prenylamine can be very effectively treated with temporary pacing [109, 110]. Prenylamine prolonged the ventricular refractoriness and repolarization, as well as decreasing the slow conduction in ischemically damaged myocardium, which accounts for its proarrhythmic potency [111].

Terodiline

Terodiline, an antispasmodic agent used to treat urinary incontinence, was withdrawn in the UK following 69 reported cases of serious arrhythythmias. Fourteen of these patients had sudden death and the remaining 55 patients had non-fatal arrhythmias including 37 patients with ventricular tachyarrhythmia, of which 24 were due to TdP [112]. It is now clear that the proarrhythmic effect of terodiline is a consequence of the blockade of I_{Kr} current [113], which occurs in a concentration-dependent manner.

Potential cardio-toxicity of β-2 adrenoceptor agonists?

In the last two decades, 2 case-control studies reported that inhaled fenoterol may have been specifically associated with the epidemic of asthma deaths in New Zealand and Canada [114, 115]. The time-trend data did not suggest a class effect of inhaled β-agonists in this epidemic. Many explanations for the association of sudden death and asthma treatment have been proposed and refuted. Among the factors that may play an important role are: the severity of asthma [116], treatment intensity [117], socioeconomic factors [118], cardiac arrhythmias (due to QT prolongation and/or changes in potassium levels) and the use of β-agonists [119, 120].

$β_2$-agonists may induce electrocardiographic changes directly, by interacting with $β_2$-receptors on the myocardium, and indirectly, by lowering extracellular potassium. It is well known that $β_2$-agonists cause an increased heart rate and have a positive inotropic effect on a failing heart. A decrease in ventricular action potential and QT interval normally occurs at high heart rates. It has been shown that a $β_1$-agonist (isoprenaline) and a $β_2$-agonist (terbutaline) shorten the myocardial action potential [121, 122]. Indeed, isoprenaline has been used for the treatment of drug-induced QT prolongation. However, when corrected for heart rate using a rate correction formula such as Bazett's formula, it was found that isoprenaline shortened the QT interval but prolonged the corrected value, known as the QTc, in a study in healthy subjects [123].

In severe acute asthma, the presence of hypoxaemia and/or hypercapnia may result in an increase in the heart rate, a fall in systemic vascular resistance, an increase in cardiac output and pulmonary artery pressure, and impaired left and right ventricular relaxation without affecting left ventricular systolic contractility [123, 125]. More importantly, acute hypoxaemia can also cause myocardial repolarization abnormalities which may have been the underlying cause of non-asthma related sudden death. Experimental studies have shown that β-agonists are lethal in dogs when the animals are hypoxic [126]. It has been hypothesized that administration of β-agonists during hypoxia may be potentially detrimental.

In a study by Bremner and colleagues, hypoxaemia alone in healthy subjects was associated with a significant increase in heart rate (8 beats/min) and QTc interval (15.6 ms). Under conditions of normoxaemia, fenoterol alone caused a significant increase in heart rate (+14.3 beats/min), systolic blood pressure (+7.7 mmHg), stroke volume (+27.7 ml), cardiac index (+1.6 1/min/m2), ejection fraction (+11.48%), and QTc interval (+32.9 ms) and a fall in QS2l (−23.2 ms) and diastolic blood pressure (−8.4 mmHg). However, when hypoxaemia and fenoterol were both present, the effects were additive (heart rate +21.9 beats/min, QTc +43.5 ms with fenoterol and hypoxaemia) [127].

Other β-agonist bronchodilator drugs that are known to cause QTc prolongation includes parenteral terbutaline from 377 ± 21 to 441 ± 39 ms in one study, but only following sequential treatment. It is important to realise that part of the reason for QTc prolongation with β-agonist may be due to its effect on hypokalaemia by stimulating cellular potassium uptake [128], which in itself is a risk factor for QTc prolongation.

The cardiovascular effects of β-agonists, however, is not a class effect and rather controversial in some β-agonists. A study by Bremner and colleagues showed that fenoterol, salbutamol and a long acting β-agonist, formoterol can all significantly increase the heart rate, QTc interval and plasma glucose, while decreasing diastolic blood pressure and plasma K^+ level compared to placebo [129]. However, salbutamol and formoterol prolonged the QTc intervals to a lower degree than fenoterol [129]. Formoterol and fenoterol caused a similar maximum reduction in plasma K^+ levels, greater than that due to salbutamol. Nevertheless, formoterol is a more selective β-agonist than fenoterol, and has similar cardiovascular effects to salbutamol when inhaled repeatedly by normal volunteers.

The effect of formoterol on QT prolongation is rather mixed. Totterman and colleagues demonstrated that at daily doses of 72 mcg and 120 mcg, formoterol was systemically less potent than 6 mg and 10 mg of terbutaline respectively on heart rate, QTc interval and serum K^+ level [130]. At very high dose of 120 mcg (5 to 10 times the recommended therapeutic dose), the effects of formoterol on heart rate, QTc interval, and plasma K^+ were small and had no clinical consequences [131]. The mean maximum increase of heart rate and QTc interval were 25.8 bpm and 25 ms at 6 hours respectively. Pulse and QTc values returned to baseline or close to baseline values at 24 h or before. K^+ levels in plasma decreased in eight out of 12 subjects; the lowest mean value was 3.53 mmol at 2 h post-dose. By 8 h post-dose, all values had returned to within the normal ranges [131].

In patients with mild to moderate asthma Burgess showed that formoterol had a dose-dependent effect on heart rate, blood pressure, electromechanical systole (QS2l), QTc interval, and plasma K^+ level. [132]. At a high dose of 96 mcg, formoterol increased the heart rate by 9 bpm, the systolic blood pressure by 4 mmHg and the QTc interval by 17 ms but decreased the diastolic BP by 3 mmHg, QS2l by 11 ms, plasma K^+ by 0.5 mmol/l and blood glucose by 2.6 mmol/l 9 hours after giving medication. The decrease in electromechanical systole indicates an increase in myocardial oxygen consumption. The increase in the QTc interval is probably clinically significant especially if the patient were to receive a high dose of formoterol whilst being profoundly hypoxaemic.

However, In a small study of 48 patients with bronchoconstriction randomized to receive formoterol (90 mcg delivered dose; 120 mcg metered dose) or terbutaline (10 mg) as well as intravenous prednisolone and oxygen, no significant effects on QTc intervals were observed before and after treatment in both treatment groups [133]. Indeed, formoterol appeared to have a wide cardiac safety margin such that if a patient happened to use extra doses of formoterol (up to total daily metered dose of 120 mcg), the QTc interval only prolonged from 415 ms at baseline to 432 ms on day 2 of treatment, and its effect was significantly less than that from a daily dose of 10 mg terbutaline [134], consistent with the mean maximum increase of 25 ms at 6 hours reported by Lecaillon et al. [131].

In the high dose studies carried out by Astra-Zeneca where formoterol 54 μg or more was given to asthmatic patients or healthy subjects, there was no consistent dose response pattern, e.g., no consistently greater prolongation after a high dose than after a low dose in the same subject. There was also no inter-patient or intra-patient consistency in terms of the time after drug administration and the greatest QTc prolongation. While there were sporadic cases of marked QT prolongation (>500 ms) or change in QTc interval (>60 ms) with high dose formoterol, the incidence did not appear to be different from what was seen after similar doses of other β_2-agonists such as terbutaline, salbutamol or salmeterol. Furthermore, despite the apparent sporadic marked QT prolongation in these studies, to date no case reports of TdP have ever been documented with β-agonists used in asthmatic patients including salbutamol and salmeterol. It is important to note that while the selection of patients with drug-induced ΔQTc > 60 ms potentially removed the possibility of spontaneous QTc variability as a cause of QT prolongation in these subjects since the variability in QTc interval in individual healthy male volunteers measured under stable conditions is approximately 75 ms, the QTc interval can still vary and exceed 500 ms spontaneously due to intra-individual variability [135].

Other β-agonists such as salbutamol has also increased the QT interval, particularly in patients with coronary heart disease [136]. In addition, salbutamol has significantly increased QT dispersion in both controls (by 48 ms) and patients with coronary artery disease (by 38 ms) [136].

Similarly, salmeterol, another long-acting β-agonist has not been shown to have any effect on the QTc interval in some studies [137, 138, 139] but in others, salmeterol has caused a dose-dependent increase in heart rate and QTc interval and a decrease in potassium level [140]. The relative dose potency of salmeterol compared with salbutamol for changes from baseline was 7.1 (95% Cl 3.9 to 14.4) for the QTc interval and 8.2 (95% Cl 5.7 to 12.6) for plasma potassium concentration. The effect on albuterol on ventricular repolarization has been rather ambiguous and unknown at the present time.

It is clear that the current evidence has not established a causal-relationship between the use of β-agonists and cardiac arrhythmia as the mechanism of sudden cardiac death. Apart from fenoterol, especially in the presence of severe hypoxaemia and the sequential use of parenteral terbutaline, other β-agonists have only demonstrated a small effect on prolonging ventricular repolarization with no clear clinical significance. Furthermore, so far there has been no documented report in the literature on an association between the use of β-agonists and TdP specifically. There is also a lack of cellular evidence on the effect of β-agonists on delayed rectifier I_{Kr} potassium channel and the available evidence on other potassium channel such as I_{Ks} is contradictory and confusing. In an experimental model of congenital LQT1 syndrome where there was a deficiency of I_{Ks} potassium channel, the addition of beta-adrenergic stimulation with isoprenaline augmented the residual I_{Ks} current in epicardial and endocardial cells but not in M cells, in which I_{Ks} is intrinsically weak and predisposed to the development of TdP by increasing the transmural dispersion of repolarization [141]. However, *in vivo* and cellular electrophysiological experiments in canine model showed that beta-adrenergic receptor stimulation with isoprenaline increased and accelerated I_{Ks} activation and shorten the action potential instead [142]. Indeed, during I_{Kr} block by other drugs, stimulation of the I_{Ks} channel with isoprenaline limits repolarization instability by time-dependent activation [142]. Thus, while there have been reports of sudden cardiac and noncardiac deaths with the use of β-agonists, there have been many confounding factors contributing to the cause of deaths in these cases and the mechanism is far from clear.

Asthma and the risk of cardiac events in high risk patients with congenital long QT syndrome

In high risk patients with congenital long QT syndrome, the website on QT prolonging drugs operated by the Arizona Center for Education and Research on Therapeutics [143] advised that albuterol and terbutaline should be avoided in these patients. It also advised that salmeterol may be associated with TdP but no substantial evidence presently supports this conclusion. Such cautionary advice is understandable given the fact that at a cellular level, β-adrenergic stimulation with isoproterenol and epinephrine induces TdP by increasing the transmural dispersion of repolarization in LQTS 1 and LQTS 2 although paradoxically suppresses TdP in LQT3 forms of the congenital long QT syndrome [144, 145].

The association between fenoterol and risk of death from asthma has been well established. However, the link between other β-agonists and death or drug-related arrhythmias in asthmatic patients is far from clear. Current clinical evidence, epidemiological studies and post-marketing surveillance do not support such a link. Although heart rate increases, QT shortening and QTc prolongation have been documented with β-agonists, the crucial QTc data have only been expressed in terms of the Bazett correction. This is known to lead to artificial prolongation of the QTc interval when tachycardia is present. Importantly there have been no case reports of TdP in association with β-agonist use in asthmatic patients, even with underlying long QT syndrome. When considering the putative arrhythmogenic potential of QT prolongation with inhaled β$_2$-agonists, the presence of associated tachycardia would tend to protect against TdP since the arrhythmia is classically more usually associated with bradycardia. Caution should probably be expressed when considering the use of β-agonists in certain high-risk patients with type 1 and type 2 congenital long QT syndromes, where β-adrenergic stimulation appears to be potentially arrhythmogenic. However, despite approximately 30 years experience with β$_2$-agonists, often administered at very high doses to critically ill patients, there is no established causal relationship or link between the QTc prolongation seen with drugs of this class and a risk for the development of ventricular arrhythmias.

Arsenic Trioxide

Arsenic trioxide has increasingly been used for relapsed acute promyelocytic leukemia. However, it is known to have severe effect on ventricular repolarization. Incidence of QT prolongation and TdP have been reported [146, 147, 148, 149]. In one study, the incidence of QT prolongation was reported to be around 63% [147]. In another study [148], prolonged QT intervals developed in 38 patients (26 patients had intervals ≥500 ms). Compared with baseline, the QTc interval was prolonged by 30 to 60 milliseconds in 36.6% of treatment courses, and by more than 60 milliseconds in 35.4% of patients. In patients receiving multiple courses, QTc intervals returned to pretreatment levels before the second course, signifying that arsenic trioxide does not permanently prolong the QT interval.

Conclusion

The list of noncardiac drugs that can cause QT prolongation and/or TdP will continue to grow. Rapidly expanding knowledge on ion channel kinetics and structure, and the molecular and genetic lesions involved in arrhythmogenesis in conditions such as the congenital long QT syndrome, has helped in the understanding of the mechanism of drug-induced proarrhythmia. Regulatory activities have increased awareness and detection of QT-prolonging effects of newer drugs, particularly those of the same pharmacological class or chemical structure. The risk of TdP is generally small but variable. The present approach to quantify such risk with clinical trial is unlikely to identify the risks as the number exposed is not large enough.

Clinical evaluations remain the cornerstone for assessing arrhythmogenic potential and the cardiac effects of any new drug before approval. Finally, postmarketing surveillance is also important in monitoring spontaneous adverse cardiac effects.

References

1 Trinkle R. Comment: syncopal episodes associated with cisapride. *Ann Pharmacother* 1999; 33 (2): 251.
2 Brans S, Murray WA, Hirsh IB, Palmer JP. Long QT syndrome during high-dose cisapride. *Arch Intern Med* 1995; 155 (7): 765–8.
3 Hoover CA, Carmichael JK, Nolan PE Jr, Marcus FI. Cardiac arrest associated with combination of cisapride and itraconazole therapy. *J Cardiovasc Pharmacol Ther* 1996; 1 (3): 255–8.
4 Wysowski DK, Bacsanyi J. Cisapride and fatal arrhythmia. *New Engl J Med* 1996; 335: 290–1.
5 Brans S, Murray WA, Hirsch IB, Palmer JP. Long QT syndrome during high-dose cisapride. *Arch Int Med* 1995; 155: 765–8.
6 Bedford TA, Rowbotham DJ. Cisapride. Drug interactions of clinical significance. *Drug Saf* 1996; 15 (3): 167–75.
7 Thomas AR, Chan LN, Bauman JL, Olopade CO. Prolongation of the QT interval related to cisapride–diltiazem interaction. *Pharmacotherapy* 1998; 18 (2): 381–5.
8 Lewin MB, Bryant RM, Fenrich AL, Grifka RG. Cisapride-induced long QT interval. *J Pediatr* 1996; 128: 279–81.
9 Olsson S, Edwards IR. Tachycardia during cisapride treatment. *Br Med J* 1992; 305: 748749.
10 Drolet B, Khalifa M, Daleau P, Hamelin BA, Turgeon J. Block of the rapid component of the delayed rectifier potassium current by the prokinetic agent cisapride underlies drug-related lengthening of the QT interval. *Circulation*, 1998; 20: 204–10.
11 Carlsson L, Amos GJ, Andersson B, Drews L, Duker G, Wadstedt G. Electrophysiological characteristics of the prokinetic agents cisapride and mosapride *in vivo* and *in vitro*: implication for proarrhythmic potential? *J Pharmacol Exp Ther*, 1997; 282 (1): 220–7.
12 Hanson R, Browne G, Fasher B, Mcaskill M, Moroney P, Hawker R. Cisapride-induced prolonged QT interval. too much of a good thing. *J Pediatr* 1997; 130 (1): 164–6.
13 Bedu A, Lupoglazoff JM, Faure C, Denjoy I, Casasoprana A, Aujard Y. Cisapride high dosage and long QT interval. *J Pediatr* 1997; 130 (1): 164.
14 Valdes L, Champel V, Olivier C, Jonville-Bera AP, Autret E. Syncope with long QT interval in a 39 day-old infant treated with cisapride. *Arch Pediatr* 1997; 4 (6): 535–7.
15 Lupoglazoff JM, Bedu A, Faure C, Denjoy I, Casasoprana A, Cezard JP, Aujard Y. Long QT syndrome under cisapride in neonates and infants. *Arch Pediatr* 1997; 4 (6): 509–14.
16 Hill SL, Evangelista JK, Pizzi AM, Mobassaleh M, Fulton DR, Berul CI. Proarrhythmia associated with cisapride in children. *Pediatrics* 1998; 101: 1053–6.
17 Khongphatthanayothin A, Lane J, Thomas D, Yen L, Chang D, Bubolz B. Effects of cisapride on QT interval in children. *J Pediatr* 1998; 133 (1): 51–6.
18 Lupoglazoff JM, Bedu A, Faure C. Long QT syndrome under cisapride in neonates and infants. *Arch Pediatr* 1997; 4: 509–14.

19 Guala A, Pastore G, Licardi G, Noe G, Zolezzi F. Effects of cisapride on QT interval in infants: a prospective study. *J Pediatr* 1997; 130 (4): 679–80.

20 Levine A, Fogelman R, Sirota L, Zangen Z, Shamir R, Dinari G. QT interval in children and infants receiving cisapride. *Pediatrics* 1998; 101 (3): e9.

21 Khoshoo V, Edell D, Clarke R. Effect of cisapride on the QT interval in infants with gastroesophageal reflux. *Pediatrics* 2000; 105 (2): e24.

22 CSM/MCA. Cisapride (Prepulsid) withdrawn. *Current Problems Pharmacovigilance* 2000; 26: 1–2.

23 Wysowski DK, Corken A, Gallo-Torres H, Talarico L, Rodriguez EM. Postmarketing reports of QT prolongation and ventricular arrhythmia in association with cisapride and Food and Drug Administration regulatory actions. *Am J Gastroenterol* 2001; 96 (6): 1698–703.

24 Iglesias E, Esteban E, Zabala S, Gascon A. Tiapride-induced torsade de pointes. *Am J Med* 2000; 109 (6): 509.

25 Kii Y, Ito T. Effects of 5HT4-receptor agonists, cisapride, mosapride citrate, and zacopride, on cardiac action potentials in guinea pig isolated papillary muscles. *J Cardiovasc Pharmacol* 1997; 29 (5): 670–5.

26 Drici MD, Ebert SN, Wang WX, Rodriguez I, Liu XK, Whitfield BH, Woosley RL. Comparison of tegaserod (HTF 919) and its main human metabolite with cisapride and erythromycin on cardiac repolarization in the isolated rabbit heart. *J Cardiovasc Pharmacol* 1999; 34 (1): 82–8.

27 Bruera E, Villamayor R, Roca E, Barugel M, Tronge J, Chacon R. QT interval prolongation and ventricular fibrillation with i. *V Domperidone Cancer Treat Rep* 1986; 70 (4): 545–6.

28 Osborne RJ, Slevin ML, Hunter RW, Hamer J. Cardiac arrhythmias during cytotoxic chemotherapy: role of domperidone. *Hum Toxicol* 1985; 4 (6): 617–26.

29 Cameron HA, Reyntjens AJ, Lake-Bakaar G. Cardiac arrest after treatment with intravenous domperidone. *BMJ* 1985; 290 (6462): 160.

30 Quinn N, Parkes D, Jackson G, Upward J. Cardiotoxicity of domperidone. *Lancet* 1985; 2 (8457): 724.

31 Osborne RJ, Slevin ML, Hunter RW, Hamer J. Cardiotoxicity of intravenous domperidone. *Lancet* 1985; 2 (8451): 385.

32 Roussak JB, Carey P, Parry H. Cardiac arrest after treatment with intravenous domperidone. *BMJ* 1984; 289: 1579.

33 Giaccone G, Berletto O, Calciati A. Two sudden deaths during prophylactic antiemetic treatment with high doses of domperidone and methylprednisolone. *Lancet* 1984; 2: 1336–7.

34 Joss RA, Goldhirsh A, Brunner KW, Galeazzi RL. Sudden death in a cancer patient on high dose domperidone. *Lancet* 1982; 1 (8279): 1019.

35 Drolet B, Rousseau G, Daleau P, Cardinal R, Turgeon J. Domperidone should not be considered a no-risk alternative to cisapride in the treatment of gastrointestinal motility disorders. *Circulation* 2000; 102: 1883–5.

36 Kamiya K, Venkatesh N, Singh BN. Acute and chronic effect of ketanserin on the electrophysiologic properties of isolated rabbit ventricular myocardium: particular reference to repolarization. *Am Heart J* 1988; 115: 1222–8.

37 Zaza A, Malfatto G, Rosen MR. Electrophysiologic effects of ketanserin on canine Purkinje fibers, ventricular myocardium and intact heart. *J Pharmacol Exp Ther* 1989; 250 (1): 397–405.

38 Zhang ZH, Follmer CH, Sing BN. Block of rapid delayed rectifier (IKr) by ketanserin in guinea pig ventricular myocytes. *Circulation* 1992; 86 (Suppl. I): I-694.

39 Zhang Z-H, Boutjdir M, El-Sherif N. Ketanserin inhibits depolarization-activated outward potassium current in rat ventricular myocytes. *Cir Res* 1994; 75: 711–21.

40 Arfiero S, Ometto R, Vincenzi M. Prolongation of the QT interval and torsades de pointes caused by ketanserin. *G Ital Cardiol* 1990; 20: 869–72.

41 Aldariz AE, Romero H, Baroni M, Baglivo H, Esper RJ. QT prolongation and torsades de pointes ventricular tachycardia produced by ketanserin. *Pacing Clin Electrophysiol* 1986; 9: 836–41.

42 Vandermotten M, Verhaeghe R, De Geest H. Ventricular arrhythmias and QT prolongation during therapy with ketanserin: report of a case. *Acta Cardiol* 1989; 44 (5): 431–7.

43 Stott DJ, Robertson JI, McLenachan JM, Ball SG. Effects of short-term ketanserin treatment on the QT interval and vagal function in healthy subjects. *J Auton Pharmacol* 1989; 9 (1): 45–51.

44 Anonymous. Prevention of atherosclerotic complications: controlled trial of ketanserin. Prevention of atherosclerotic complications with ketanserin trial group. *BMJ* 1989; 298 (6671): 424–30.

45 Zehender M, Meinertz T, Hohnloser S, Geibel A, Hartung J, Seiler KU, Just H. Incidence and clinical relevance of QT prolongation caused by the new selective serotonin antagonist ketanserin. *Multicenter Ketanserin Res Group Clin Physiol Biochem* 1990; 8 (Suppl. 3): 90–100.

46 Cameron HA, Waller PC, Ramsay LE. Prolongation of the QT interval by ketanserin. *Postgrad Med J* 1988; 64 (748): 112–7.

47 Marshall FN, Lewis JE. Sensitization to epinephrine-induced ventricular fibrillation produced by probucol in dogs. *Toxicol Appl Pharmacol* 1973; 24: 594–602.

48 Troendle G, Gueriguian J, Sobel J, Johnson M. Probucol and the QT interval. *Lancet* 1982; 1 (8282): 1179.

49 Miettinen TA, Huttunen JK, Kuusi T, Kumlin T, Mattila S, Naukkarinen V, Strandberg T. Clinical experience with probucol with special emphasis on mode of action and long-term treatment. *Artery* 1982; 10: 35–43.

50 Molello JA, Gerbig CG, Robinson VB. Toxicity of [4, 4'-(isopropyline-dithio) bis (2,6-di-t-butylphenol)], probucol, in mice, rats, dogs and monkeys: demonstration of species-specific phenomenon. *Toxicol Appl Pharmacol* 1973; 24: 590–3.

51 Matsuhashi H, Onodera S, Kawamura Y, Hasebe N, Kohmura C, Yamashita H, Tobise K. Probucol-induced QT prolongation and torsades de pointes. *Jpn J Med* 1989; 28 (5): 612–5.

52 Kajinami K, Takekoshi N, Mabuchi H. Propranolol for probucol-induced QT prolongation with polymorphic ventricular tachycardia. *Lancet* 1993; 341 (8837): 124–5.

53 Tamura M, Ueki Y, Ohtsuka E, Oribe M, Seita M, Oribe K, Ito M. Probucol-induced QT prolongation and syncope. *Jpn Circ J* 1994; 58 (5): 374–7.

54 Ohya Y, Kumamoto K, Abe I, Tsubota Y, Fujishima M. Factors related to QT interval prolongation during probucol treatment. *Eur J Clin Pharmacol* 1993; 45: 47–52.

55 McCaughan D. Probucol and the QT interval. *Lancet* 1982; 2 (8290): 161.

56 Browne KF, Prystowsky EN, Heger JJ, Cerimele BJ, Fineberg N, Zipes DP. Prolongation of the QT interval induced by probucol: demonstration of a method for determining QT interval change induced by a drug. *Am Heart J* 1984; 107: 680–4.

57 Troendle G, Gueriguian J, Sobel J, Johnson M. Probucol and the QT interval. *Lancet* 1982; 1: 1179.

58 Dujovne CA, Atkins F, Wong B, DeCoursey S, Krehbiel P, Chernoff SB. Electrocardiographic effects of probucol. A controlled prospective clinical trial. *Eur J Clin Pharmacol* 1984; 26: 735–9.

59 Hodak SP, Moubarak JB, Rodriguez I, Gelfand MC, Alijani MR, Tracy CM. QT prolongation and near fatal cardiac arrhythmia after intravenous tacrolimus administration: a
   case report. *Transplantation* 1998; 66 (4): 535–7.

60 Johnson MC, So S, Marsh JW, Murphy AM. QT prolongation and torsades de pointes
   after administration of FFK506. *Transplantation* 1992; 53 (4): 929–30.

61 Minematsu T, Ohtani H, Sato H, Iga I. Sustained QT prolongation induced by tacrolimus
   in guinea pigs. *Life Sci* 1999; 65 (14): 197–202.

62 Kupferschmidt H, Meier CH, Sulzer M, Meier PJ, Buhler H. Clinico-pharmacological
   case (2). Bradycardia and ventricular tachycardia of the torsades de pointes type as a
   side-effect of vasopression: 3 case reports. *Schweiz Rundsch Med Prax* 1996; 85 (11): 340–3.

63 Stein LB, Dabezies MA, Silverman M, Bronzena SC. Fatal torsades de pointes occurring
   in a patient receiving intravenous vesopressin and nitroglycerin. *J Clin Gastroenterol* 1992;
   15 (2): 171–4.

64 Klein GJ. Vasopressin, "torsades de pointes", and QT syndrome. *Ann Intern Med* 1980; 93
   (3): 511–2.

65 Mauro VF, Bingle JF, Ginn SM, Jafri FM. Torsades de pointes in a patient receiving
   intravenous vasopressin. *Crit Care Med* 1988; 16 (2): 200–1.

66 Faigel DO, Metz DC, Kochman ML. Torsades de pointes complicating the treatment
   bleeding esophageal varices: association with neuroleptics, vasopression, and electrolyte
   imbalance. *Am J Gastroenterol* 1995; 90 (5): 822–4.

67 Celiker A, Brugada P. Adenosine induced torsades de pointes in long QT syndrome.
   (Abstract) XIIth Meeting Belgiam Working Group Cardiac Pacing and Electrophysiology, 1992.

68 Celiker A, Tokel K, Cil E, Ozkutlu S, Ozme S. Adenosine induced torsades de pointes in a
   child with long QT syndrome. *Pacing Clin Electrophysiol* 1994; 17 (1): 1814–7.

69 Wesley RC, Turnquest P. Torsades de pointe after intravenous adenosine in the presence
   of prolonged QT syndrome. *Am Heart J* 1992; 123 (3): 794–6.

70 Harrington GR, Froelich EG. Adenosine-induced torsades de pointes. *Chest* 1993; 103 (4):
   1299–301.

71 Romer M, Candinas R. Adenosine-induced nonsustained polymorphic ventricular
   tachycardia. *Eur Heart J* 1994; 15 (2): 281–2.

72 Smith JR, Goldberger JJ, Kadish AH. Adenosine induced polymorphic ventricular tachycardia in adults without structural heart disease. *Pacing Clin Electrophysiol* 1997; 20 (1):
   743–5.

73 Povoa R, Cardoso SH, Luno Filho B, Ferreira Filho C, Ferreira M, Ferreira C. Organophosphate poisoning and myocardial necrosis. *Arr Bras Cardiol* 1997; 68 (5): 377–80.

74 Wang MH, Tseng CD, Bair SY. QT interval prolongation and pleomorphic ventricular
   tachyarrhythmia ("torsade de pointes") in organophosphate poisoning: report of a case.
   Hum Exp Toxicol 1998; 17 (10): 587–90.

75 Wazakowska-Kaplon B, Janion M, Konstantynowicz H, Buda S, Gutkowski W. Long QT
   syndrome after organophosphate insecticide poisoning. *Kardiol Pol* 1992; 36 (4): 220–3.

76 Kiss Z, Fezekas T. Arrhythmias in organophosphate poisonings. *Acta Cardiol* 1979; 34 (5):
   323–30.

77 Chuang FR, Jang SW, Lin JL, Chern MS, Chen JB, Hsu KT. QTc prolongation indicates a
   poor prognosis in patients with organophosphate poisoning. *Am J Emerg Med* 1996; 14
   (5): 451–3.

78 Nanji AA, Filipenko JD. Asystole and ventricular fibrillation associated with cocaine
   intoxication. *Chest* 1984; 85: 132–3.

79 Schrem SS, Belsky P, Schwartzman D, Slater W. Cocaine-induced torsades de pointes in a patient with the idiopathic long QT syndrome. *Am Heart J* 1990; 120 (4): 980–4.

80 Gamoras GA, Monir G, Plunkitt K, Gursoy S, Dreifus LS. Cocaine abuse: repolarization abnormalities and ventricular arrhythmias. *Am J Med Sci* 2000; 320 (1): 9–12.

81 Clarkson CW, Chang C, Stolfi A, George WJ, Yamasaki S, Pickoff S. Electrophysiological effects of high cocaine concentrations on intact canine heart. Evidence for modulation by both heart rate and autonomic nervous system. *Circulation* 1993; 87: 950–62.

82 Temesy-Armos PN, Fraker TD Jr, Brewster PS, Wilkerson RD. The effects of cocaine on cardiac electrophysiology in conscious unsedated dogs. *J Cardiovasc Pharmacol* 1992; 19 (6): 883–91.

83 Jain A, Jenkins MG. Intracoronary electrocardiogram during torsade des pointes secondary to intracoronary papaverine. *Cathet Cardiovasc Diagn* 1989; 18 (4): 255–7.

84 Kern MJ, Deligonul U, Serota H, Gudipati C, Buckingham T. Ventricular arrhythmia due to intracoronary papaverine. analysis of QT intervals and coronary vasodilatory reserve. *Cathet Cardiovasc Diagn* 1990; 19 (4): 229–36.

85 Vrolix M, Piessens J, De Geest H. Torsades de pointes after intracoronary papaverine. *Eur Heart J* 1991; 12 (2): 273–6.

86 Zhang X, Shen W, Cai X, Zheng A. Polymorphous ventricular tachycardia after intracoronary papaverine: a report of three cases. *Chin Med Sci J* 1993; 8 (4): 248–9.

87 Talman CL, Winniford MD, Rossen JD, Simonetti I, Kienzle MG, Marcus ML. Polymorphous ventricular tachycardia: a side-effect of intracoronary papaverine. *J Am Coll Cardiol* 1990; 15 (2): 275–8.

88 Inoue T, Asahi S, Takayanagi K, Morooka S, Takabatake Y. QT prolongation and possibility of ventricular arrhythmias after intracoronary papaverine. *Cardiology* 1994; 84 (1): 9–13.

89 Pinter A, Dorian P, Newman D. Cesium-induced torsades de pointes. *N Engl J Med* 2002; 346 (5): 383–4.

90 Coumel P. Safety of bepridil: from review of the European data. *Am J Cardiol* 1992; 69: 75D–78D.

91 Makkar RR, Fromm BS, Steinman RT, Meissner MD, Lehmann MH. Female gender as a risk factor for torsades de pointes associated with cardiovascular drugs. *JAMA* 1993; 270: 2590–7.

92 Gill A, Flaim SF, Damiano BP, Sit SP, Brannan MD. Pharmacology of bepridil. *Am J Cardiol* 1992; 69(11): 11D–16D.

93 Singh BN. Bepridil therapy: guidelines for patient selection and monitoring of therapy. *Am J Cardiol* 1992; 69(11): 79D–85D.

94 Weiss RJ, Schulman P, Marriott T *et al*. Efficacy and safety of bepridil in chronic stable angina pectoris refractory to nifedipine. *Am J Ther* 1994; 1(4): 276–80.

95 Narahara KA, Singh BN, Karliner JS, Corday SR, Hossack KF. Bepridil hydrochloride compared with placebo in patients with stable angina pectoris. *Am J Cardiol* 1992; 69(11): 37D–42D.

96 Singh BN. Safety profile of bepridil determined from clinical trials in chronic stable angina in the United States. *Am J Cardiol* 1992; 69(11): 68D–74D.

97 Coumel P. Safety of bepridil: from review of the European data. *Am J Cardiol* 1992; 69(11): 75D–78D.

98 Funck-Brentano C, Coudray P, Planellas J, Motte G, Jaillon P. Effects of bepridil and diltiazem on ventricular repolarization in angina pectoris. *Am J Cardiol* 1990; 66(10): 812–17.

99 Yoshiga Y, Shimizu A, Yamagata T *et al*. Beta-blocker decreases the increase in QT dispersion and transmural dispersion of repolarization induced by bepridil. *Circ J* 2002; 66(11): 1024–8.

100 Chouabe C, Drici MD, Romey G, Barhanin J. Effects of calcium channel blockers on cloned cardiac K+ channels I_{Kr} and I_{Ks}. *Therapie* 2000; 55(1): 195–202.

101 Osaka T, Kodama I, Toyama J, Yamada K. Effects of bepridil on ventricular depolarization and repolarization of rabbit isolated hearts with particular reference to its possible proarrhythmic properties. *Br J Pharmacol* 1988; 93(4): 775–80.

102 Glaser S, Steinbach M, Opitz C, Wruck U, Kleber FX. Torsades de pointes caused by Mibefradil. *Eur J Heart Fail* 2001; 3(5): 627–30.

103 Chouabe C, Drici MD, Romey G, Barhanin J, Lazdunski M. HERG and KvLQT1/IsK, the cardiac K+ channels involved in long QT syndromes are targets for calcium channel blockers. *Mol Pharmacol* 1998; 54(4): 695–703.

104 Normand JP, Kahn JC, Mialet G, Bardet G, Bourdarias JP, Mathivat A. "Torsades de pointe" induced or stimullated by prenylamine. Apropos of 4 cases. *Ann Cardiol Angeiol (Paris)* 1974; 23(6): 527–33.

105 Kadiwar RM, MacMahon B. Prenylamine induced torsade de pointes. *Ir Med J* 1990; 83(4): 163.

106 Mohr R. Torsades de pointe with prenylamine. *Lancet* 1986; 2(8517): 1218.

107 Makkar RR, Fromm BS, Steinman RT, Meissner MD, Lehmann MH. Female gender as a risk factor for torsades de pointes associated with cardiovascular drugs. *JAMA* 1993; 270(21): 2590–7.

108 Oakley D, Jennings K, Puritz R, Krikler D, Chamberlain D. The effect of prenylamine on the QT interval of the resting electrocardiogram in patients with angina pectoris. *Postgrad Med J* 1980; 56(661): 753–6.

109 Grenadier E, Keidar S, Alpan G, Marmor A, Palant A. Prenylamine-induced ventricular tachycardia and syncope controlled by ventricular pacing. *Br Heart J* 1980; 44(3): 330–4.

110 DiSegni E, Klein HO, David D, Libhaber C, Kaplinsky E. Overdrive pacing in quinidine syncope and other long QT-interval syndromes. *Arch Intern Med* 1980; 140(8): 1036–40.

111 Aidonidis I, Egel E, Hilbel T, Kuebler W, Brachmann J. Effects of prenylamine and AQ-A 39 on reentrant ventricular arrhythmias induced during the late myocardial infarction period in conscious dogs. *J Cardiovasc Pharmacol* 1993; 22(3): 401–7.

112 CSM/MCA. Terodiline. *Current Problems in Pharmacovigilance* 1991; 32: 1.

113 Jones SE, Ogura T, Shuba LM, McDonald TF. Inhibition of the rapid component of the delayed-rectifier K+ current by therapeutic concentrations of the antispasmodic agent terodiline. *Br J Pharmacol* 1998; 125: 1138–43.

114 Pearce N, Beasley R, Crane J, Burgess C, Jackson R. End of the New Zealand asthma mortality epidemic. *Lancet.* 1995; 345(8941): 41–44.

115 Spitzer WO, Suissa S, Ernst P *et al.* The use of beta-agonists and the risk of death and near death from asthma. *N Engl J Med* 1992; 326(8): 501–6.

116 Barriot P, Riou B. Prevention of fatal asthma. *Chest* 1987; 92: 460–6.

117 Jalaludin BB, Smith MA, Chey T *et al.* Risk factors for asthma deaths: a population-based, case-control study. *Aust NZ J Public Health* 1999; 23: 595–600.

118 Corn B, Hamrung G, Ellis A *et al.* Patterns of asthma death and near-death in an inner city tertiary care teaching hospital. *J Asthma* 1995; 32: 405–12.

119 Beasley R, Burgess C, Pearce N *et al.* Confounding by severity does not explain the association between fenoterol and asthma death. *Clin Exp Allergy* 1994; 24: 660–8.

120 Pearce N, Grainger J, Atkinson M *et al.* Case-control study of prescribed fenoterol and death from asthma in New Zealand, 1977–81. *Thorax* 1990; 45: 170–5.

121 Newman D, Dorian P, Feder-Elituv R. Isoproterenol antagonizes drug-induced prolongation of action potential duration in humans. *Can J Physiol Pharmacol* 1993; 71: 755–60.

122 Arlock P. Actions of prenalterol, a new cardioselective beta1-agonist, terbutaline and isoprenaline on electrophysiological and mechanical parameters of guinea pig atrial and papillary muscles. *Acta Pharmacol Toxicol (Copenh)* 1982; 51(1): 12–19.

123 Shimizu W, Ohe T, Kurita T, Shimomura K. Differential response of QTU interval to exercise, isoproterenol, and atrial pacing in patients with congenital long QT syndrome. *Pacing Clin Electrophysiol* 1991; 14: 1966–70.

124 Cargill RI, Kiely DG, Lipworth BJ. Left ventricular systolic performance during acute hypoxemia. *Chest* 1995; 108: 899–902.

125 Cargill RI, Kiely DG, Lipworth BJ. Adverse effects of hypoxaemia on diastolic filling in humans. *Clin Sci* 1995; 89: 165–9.

126 Collins IWE, McDevitt DG, Shanks RG et al. The cardiotoxicity of isoprenaline during hypoxia. *Br J Pharmacol* 1969; 36: 35–45.

127 Bremner P, Burgess CD, Crane J et al. Cardiovascular effects of fenoterol under conditions of hypoxaemia. *Thorax* 1992; 47: 814–17.

128 Braden GL, von Oeyen PT, Germain MJ, Watson DJ, Haag BL. Ritodrine- and terbutaline-induced hypokalemia in preterm labor: mechanisms and consequences. *Kidney Int* 1997; 51(6): 1867–75.

129 Brenmer P, Woodman K, Burgess C, Crane J, Purdie G, Pearce N, Beasley R. A comparison of the cardiovascular and metabolic effects of formoterol, salbutamol and fenoterol. *Eur Respir J* 1993; 6(2): 204–10.

130 Totterman KJ, Huhti L, Sutinen E et al. Tolerability to high doses of formoterol and terbutaline via Turbuhaler for 3 days in stable asthmatic patients. *Eur Respir J* 1998; 12(3): 573–9.

131 Lecaillon JB, Kaiser G, Palmisano M, Morgan J, Della Cioppa G. Pharmacokinetics and tolerability of formoterol in healthy volunteers after a single high dose of Foradil dry powder inhalation via Aerolizer. *Eur J Clin Pharmacol* 1999; 55(2): 131–8.

132 Burgess C, Ayson M, Rajasingham S, Crane J, Della Cioppa G, Till MD. The extrapulmonary effects of increasing doses of formoterol in patients with asthma. *Eur J Clin Pharmacol* 1998; 54(2): 141–7.

133 Malolepszy J, Boszormenyi Gagy G, Selroos O, Larsson P, Brander R. Safety of formoterol Turbuhaler® at cumulative dose of 90 μg in patients with acute bronchial obstruction. *Eur Respir J* 2001; 18: 928–34.

134 Totterman KJ, Huhti L, Sutinen E et al. Tolerability to high doses of formoterol and terbutaline via Turbuhaler for 3 days in stable asthmatic patients. *Eur Respir J* 1998; 12(3): 573–9.

135 Morganroth J, Brozovich FV, McDonald JT, Jacobs RA. Variability of the QT measurement in healthy men, with implications for selection of an abnormal QT value to predict drug toxicity and proarrhythmia. *Am J Cardiol* 1991; 67: 774–6.

136 Lowe MD, Rowland E, Brown MJ, Grace AA. B2 adrenergic receptors mediate important electrophysiological effects in human ventricular myocardium. *Heart* 2002; 86: 45–51.

137 Tunaoglu FS, Turktas I, Olgunturk R, Demirsoy S. Cardiac side effects of long-acting beta-2 agonist salmeterol in asthmatic children. *Pediatr Int* 1999; 41(1): 28–31.

138 Bagnato GF, Mileto A, Gulli S et al. Acute cardiovascular effects of salmeterol in subjects with stable bronchial asthma. *Monaldi Arch Chest Dis* 1996; 51(4): 275–8.

139 Ferguson GT, Funck-Brentano C, Fischer T, Darken P, Reisner C. Cardiovascular safety of salmeterol in COPD. *Chest* 2003; 123(6): 1817–24.

140 Bennett JA, Tattersfield AE. Time course and relative dose potency of systemic effects from salmeterol and salbutamol in healthy subjects. *Thorax* 1997; 452(5): 458–64.

141 Shimizu W, Antzelevitch C. Cellular basis for the ECG features of the LQT1 form of the long-QT syndrome: effects of beta-adrenergic agonists and antagonists and sodium channel blockers on transmural dispersion of repolarization and torsade de pointes. *Circulation* 1998; 98(21): 2314–22.

142 Volders PG, Stengl M, van Opstal JM *et al.* Probing the contribution of IKs to canine ventricular repolarization: key role for beta-adrenergic receptor stimulation. *Circulation* 2003; 107(21): 2753–60.

143 http://www.qtdrugs.org/medical-pros/drug-lists/printable-drug-list.cfm.

144 Shimizu W, Antzelevitch C. Differential effects of beta-adrenergic agonists and antagonists in LQT1, LQT2 and LQT3 models of the long QT syndrome. *J Am Coll Cardiol* 2000; 35(3): 778–86.

145 Shimizu W, Tanabe Y, Aiba T *et al.* Differential effects of beta-blockade on dispersion of repolarization in the absence and presence of sympathetic stimulation between the LQT1 and LQT2 forms of congenital long QT syndrome. *J Am Coll Cardiol* 2002; 39(12): 1984–91.

146 Ohnishi K, Yoshida H, Shigeno K *et al.* Prolongation of the QT interval and ventricular tachycardia in patients treated with arsenic trioxide for acute promyelocytic leukemia. *Ann Intern Med* 2000; 133(11): 881–5.

147 Unnikrishnan D, Dutcher JP, Varshneya N *et al.* Torsades de pointes in 3 patients with leukemia treated with arsenic trioxide. *Blood* 2001; 97(5): 1514–16.

148 Soignet SL, Frankel SR, Douer D *et al.* United States multicenter study of arsenic trioxide in relapsed acute promyelocytic leukemia. *J Clin Oncol* 2001; 19(18): 3852–60.

149 Barbey JT, Pezzullo JC, Soignet SL. Effect of arsenic trioxide on QT interval in patients with advanced malignancies. *J Clin Oncol* 2003; 21(19): 3609–15.

CHAPTER 10

Acquired long QT syndrome secondary to cardiac conditions

Myocardial infarction

An early report by Schwartz and Wolf [1] demonstrated that the QT interval is significantly prolonged after myocardial infarction (MI) compared to controls. Furthermore, the incidence of QT prolongation is more common in MI patients who had sudden death compared to survivors (57% vs. 18% and 443 ± 27 vs. 429 ± 20 ms, respectively). Among patients with previous MI, a prolonged QT interval of over 440 ms constituted a 2.16 times greater risk for sudden death. Other workers confirmed that QT prolongation after acute MI predicts ventricular fibrillation and/or tachycardia [2]. In patients who developed early ventricular tachycardia within the first 48 h of acute MI, the initial QT interval upon hospitalization was significantly longer compared with patients with only frequent premature beats (520 ± 70 ms vs. 470 ± 30 ms) and by the fifth day after the acute MI, the QT interval shortened significantly only in the ventricular tachycardia group [3]. Thus, the initial transient prolongation of ventricular repolarization facilitates and predicts complex ventricular tachyarrhythmias within the first 48 h of acute MI.

During the acute phase, patients with anterior MI had longer QT intervals compared with inferior MI, and patients with subendocardial MI had longer QT intervals than patients with full-thickness infarct, although this is generally transient [2] [Fig. 10.1]. During the chronic period, MI patients who had reinfarction had longer QT intervals. On the other hand, patients receiving beta-blockers had shorter QT intervals than those who did not [2]. The QT interval was most prolonged during the first 2 days and gradually shortened over the course of 12 months after MI [2]. However, polymorphic ventricular tachycardia occurring in the setting of acute MI was rare and appeared to be unrelated to QT prolongation, sinus bradycardia, preceding sinus pauses, or electrolyte abnormalities, but was often associated with signs or symptoms of recurrent myocardial ischemia [4]. Other workers, however, found that the QT interval did not change during transient myocardial ischaemia, regardless of previous infarction or extent of coronary artery disease [5].

In patients with acute MI, approximately 30% had prolonged QT intervals (QTc $\geq$ 440 ms). The longest QTc was observed in patients suffering from VT and/or in nonsurvivors [6]. Acute stabilization of polymorphic ventricular tachycardia could be achieved by intravenous amiodarone (despite its low risk of proarrhythmia) and/or emergency coronary revascularization [4]. The

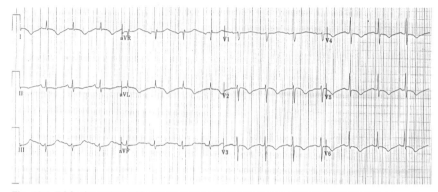

Fig. 10.1 ECG of a patient with antero-septal-lateral non-Q wave infarct. Note the QTc interval was 598 ms with morphologically abnormal T/U wave complex and prolonged offset of the repolarization.

QT interval correlated closely with left ventricular function. Patients with a prolonged QT interval, especially those with acute anterior or antero-inferior myocardial infarction, had worse left ventricular dysfunction [7].

The prolonged action potential duration after MI has been shown to be attributed to decreased density of the two outward potassium currents, I_{to}-fast (I_{to}-f) and I_{to}-slow (I_{to}-s), rather than changes in the density and/or kinetics of the L-type Ca^{2+} current. The changes in ionic current density may be related to alterations in the expression and levels of ion channel proteins [8].

Dilated cardiomyopathy and congestive heart failure

QT prolongation in patients with dilated cardiomyopathy is common [Fig. 10.2]. In one small report of 25 children with dilated cardiomyopathy, 32% of the patients had a QTc interval > 450 ms [9]. The QT interval was not related to fractional shortening or left ventricular end-diastolic dimensions [9]. At the cellular level, action potentials were markedly prolonged in the failing myocytes, as a result of reductions in Ito and I_{K1} potassium currents [10–12]. More recently, studies also showed that mRNA transcripts for both HERG gene (encoding I_{Kr}) and KV4.3 (encoding I_{to}) are reduced in the left ventricles in patients with advanced heart failure [13]. It has been shown that in patients with congestive heart failure, QT prolongation can be nearly normalized by an elevation of serum potassium level, possibly by increasing the I_{Kr} and/or I_{K1} currents independently, leading to an overall increase in repolarizing current, thus shortening the action potential duration and reversing QT prolongation [14]. Other factors that are likely to contribute to QT prolongation include modulation of ion currents by an activated autonomic nervous system and by other hormones, the presence of underlying structural heart disease or ischemia and electrolyte imbalances secondary to diuretic

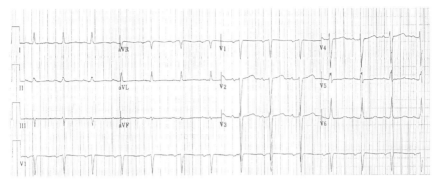

Fig. 10.2 ECG of a 30-year-old-patient with familial dilated cardiomyopathy. The ECG showed a prolonged QTc interval of 576 ms and incomplete left bundle branch block, both of which are common features of dilated cardiomyopathy.

therapy. Congestive heart failure is also a major risk factor for TdP associated with I_{Kr} blocking drugs. For instance the incidence of TdP induced by dofetilide was 2.1% among the 1511 patients with reduced left ventricular ejection fraction or clinical heart failure from both DIAMOND-MI and -CHF studies.

Hypertrophic cardiomyopathy

Although there is no known genetic association between congenital long QT syndrome and hypertrophic cardiomyopathy, QT prolongation is often seen in patients with hypertrophic cardiomyopathy [15]. The QT interval in patients with hypertrophic cardiomyopathy is not related to interventricular septal thickness [9] but there is a significant correlation between the degree of left ventricular hypertrophy expressed by the maximum wall thickness and maximum QTc [16].

Studies from St. George's Hospital showed that the QTc interval (Bazett's correction) in patients with hypertrophic cardiomyopathy was significantly prolonged compared to healthy controls (432 ± 27 vs. 404 ± 16 ms) [17,18]. There were no significant differences in the QTc interval (Bazett's and Fridericia's corrections) between high risk (sudden cardiac death and/or documented ventricular fibrillation) and low risk patients [18]. The true incidence of hypertrophic cardiomyopathy patients with prolonged QTc interval ≥ 450 ms is unknown, although in one small study it has been reported to be 24% [9]. Recently, a sophisticated algorithm that enabled the assessment of the temporal repolarization lability (defined as the ratio between QT and heart rate variability) showed that hypertrophic cardiomyopathy patients with α-myosin heavy chain gene mutations exhibited labile repolarization, and may be more at risk for sudden death [19].

Hypertension

In patients with essential hypertension, the QT interval is prolonged especially in those with left ventricular hypertrophy. In these patients, the QT interval correlated positively with left ventricular mass index and left ventricular internal diastolic dimension [20]. The longest QT intervals were detected in patients with left ventricular hypertrophy and complex ventricular arrhythmias (grade 3 and 4 ventricular arrhythmias according to a modified Lown and Wolf classification). Thus, it has been suggested that QT prolongation in patients with left ventricular hypertrophy secondary to essential hypertension may be a marker for the increased risk of arrhythmias. A QTc duration >380 ms had a sensitivity of 74% and a specificity of 89% for detecting complex ventricular arrhythmias. Long-term enalapril treatment of hypertensive patients with left ventricular hypertrophy induced marked regression of left ventricular mass and improved left ventricular systolic function and shortened QT interval, which probably reduces the likelihood of ventricular arrhythmias and improves prognosis [21]. Furthermore, in hypertensive patients with left ventricular hypertrophy, the QT interval response to changes in the RR interval is rapid and exaggerated, suggesting that the altered repolarization dynamics in these patients may make them vulnerable to serious ventricular arrhythmias [22].

Bradycardia

Although patients with complete heart block are at risk of dying from asystole, QT prolongation and TdP from bradycardia in patients with complete heart block has also been reported [23] [Figs 10.3–10.5]. Such cases illustrate the importance of assessing the QT interval in patients with atrioventricular block, and demonstrate that syncopal episodes, and possibly sudden death, in patients with complete heart block can be due to bradycardia-induced ventricular tachyarrhythmias, rather than extreme bradycardia *per se*.

Kurita *et al.* examined 14 patients with complete heart block and noted that during the acute period, patients with TdP (six patients) had significantly longer QTc intervals than those without TdP (585 $\pm$ 44.8 vs. 476 $\pm$ 58.3 ms, $P < 0.001$) [24]. Two months after pacemaker implantation, when the QT interval was rechecked after the pacemaker rate was reset from 90 or 100 bpm to 60 and 50 bpm, the QTc interval remained more prolonged in the TdP group than in those without TdP (60 bpm: 551 $\pm$ 40 vs. 503 $\pm$ 36 ms, $P < 0.005$; 50 bpm: 700 $\pm$ 46 vs. 529 $\pm$ 43 ms, $P < 0.001$). Thus patients with complete heart block and TdP had a bradycardia-sensitive repolarization abnormality, which remained after treatment with pacemaker implantation (when the heart rate was reduced <60 bpm). In a retrospective survey, the absolute QT interval ranged from 520 to 880 ms, with a mean of 680 ms, during complete heart block and at a mean heart rate of 37 bpm [25].

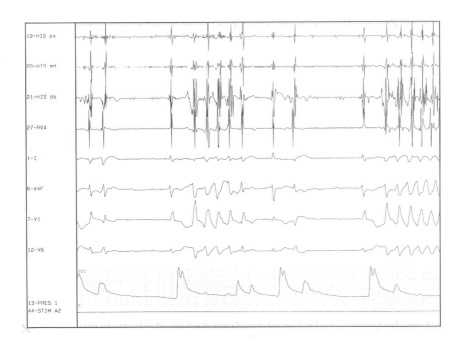

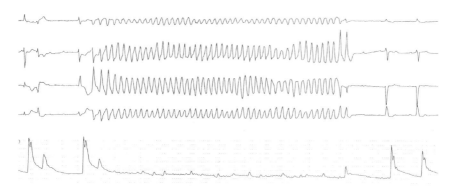

Fig. 10.3 TdP triggered by intermittent complete atrio-ventricular block in a female patient who had QT prolongation induced by sotalol (QTc = 517 ms), prescribed for the treatment for hypertension.

Bradycardia increases the amplitude of early after-depolarization and produces abnormal repolarization, thus increases the risk of TdP [26]. This applies to both patients with atrio-ventricular and sino-atrial blocks. Bradycardia produced early after-depolarizations, characterized as a distinct hump on phase 3 repolarization of the monomorphic action potentials, which was associated with marked prolongation of the QTU interval on the surface ECG. The amplitude of early after-depolarizations was bradycardia dependent,

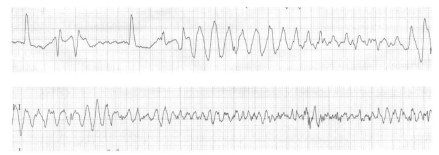

Fig. 10.4 The ECG of the same patient of Fig. 1.2, p. 3 who developed TdP leading to ventricular fibrillation secondary to bradycardia from sick sinus syndrome.

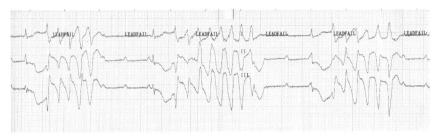

Fig. 10.5 An elderly female patient who has complete heart block developed self-terminating nonsustained TdP while having her pacemaker generator replaced. The TDP disappeared after she was paced at VVI mode.

and there was a strong correlation between the preceding RR interval and the amplitude of the early after-depolarizations [27].

Kawasaki syndrome and myocarditis

Other less common cardiac causes of acquired long QT syndrome include Kawasaki syndrome and myocarditis [28,29], including acute rheumatic carditis [30]. The reasons for QT prolongation in these conditions remain unclear. However, it is possible to speculate that QT prolongation in patients with Kawasaki syndrome may be due to the abnormal T wave morphology whereas in patients with myocarditis, it may result from the underlying congestive heart failure.

References

1 Schwartz PJ, Wolf S. QT interval prolongation as predictor of sudden death in patients with myocardial infarction. *Circulation* 1978; 57: 1074–7.
2 Ahnve S. QT interval prolongation in acute myocardial infarction. *Eur Heart J* 1985; 6: D85–95.

3 Taylor GJ, Crampton RS, Gibson RS, Stebbins PT, Waldman MT, Beller GA. Prolonged QT interval at onset of acute myocardial infarction in predicting early phase ventricular tachycardia. *Am Heart J* 1981; 102 (1): 16–24.

4 Wolfe CL, Nibley C, Bhandari A, Chatterjee K, Scheinman M. Polymorphic ventricular tachycardia associated with acute myocardial infarction. *Circulation* 1991; 84: 1543–51.

5 Kerr CR, Hacking A, Henning H. Effects of transient myocardial ischemia on the QT interval in man. *Can J Cardiol* 1987; 3 (8): 383–6.

6 Assmann I, Muller E. Prognostic significance of different QT-intervals in the body surface ECG in patients with acute myocardial infarction and in patients with acute or chronic cerebral processes. *Acta Cardiol* 1990; 45 (6): 501–4.

7 Raev D. Relationship between rate-corrected QT interval and wall motion abnormalities in the setting of acute myocardial infarction. *Int J Cardiol* 1997; 61 (1): 15–20.

8 Gidh-Jain M, Huang B, Jain P, el-Sherif N. Differential expression of voltage-gated K+ channel genes in left ventricular remodeled myocardium after experimental myocardial infarction. *Circ Res* 1996; 79 (4): 669–75.

9 Martin AB, Garson A, Perry JC. Prolonged QT interval in hypertrophic and dilated cardiomyopathy in children. *Am Heat J* 1994; 127: 64–70.

10 Beuckelmann DJ, Nabauer M, Erdmann E. Alterations of K^+-current in isolated human ventricular myocytes from patients with terminal heart failure. *Cir Res* 1993; 73: 379–85.

11 Hart G. Cellular electrophysiology in cardiac hypertrophy and failure. *Cardiovasc Res* 1994; 28: 933–46.

12 Kaab S, Nuss HB, Chiamvimonvat N, O'Rourke B, Pak PH, Kass DA, Marban E, Tomaselli GF. Ionic mechanism of action potential prolongation in ventricular myocytes from dogs with pacing-induced heart failure. *Cir Res* 1996; 78: 262–73.

13 Choy AM, Kupershmidt S, Lang CC, Pierson RN Jr, Roden DM. Regional expression of HERG and KVLQT1 in heart failure. *Circulation* 1996: 94: I–164.

14 Choy AM, Lang CC, Chomsky DM, Rayos GH, Wilson JR, Roden DM. Normalization of acquired QT prolongation in humans by intravenous potassium. *Circulation* 1997; 96: 2149–54.

15 Priori SG, Barhanin J, Hauer RN *et al.* Genetic and molecular basis of cardiac arrhythmias: impact on clinical management parts I and II. *Circulation* 1999; 99 (4): 518–28.

16 Dritsas A, Sbarouni E, Gilligan D, Nihoyannopoulos P, Oakley CM. QT-interval abnormalities in hypertrophic cardiomyopathy. *Clin Cardiol* 1992; 15 (10): 739–42.

17 Yi G, Elliott P, McKenna WJ, Prasad K, Sharma S, Guo XH, Camm AJ, Malik M. QT dispersion and risk factors for sudden cardiac death in patients with hypertrophic cardiomyopathy. *Am J Cardiol* 1998; 82: 1514–9.

18 Fei L, Slade AK, Grace AA, Malik M, Camm AJ, McKenna WJ. Ambulatory assessment of the QT interval in patients with hypertrophic cardiomyopathy: risk stratification and effect of low dose amiodarone. *Pacing Clin Electrophysiol* 1994; 17 (11 Part 2): 2222–7.

19 Atiga WL, Fananapazir L, McAreavey D, Calkins H, Berger RD. Temporal repolarization lability in hypertrophic cardiomyopathy casued by α-myosin heavy-chain gene mutations. *Circulation* 2000; 101: 1237–42.

20 Kulan K, Ural D, Komsuoglu B, Agacdiken A, Goldeli O, Komsuoglu SS. Significance of QTc prolongation on ventricular arrhythmias in patients with left ventricular hypertrophy secondary to essential hypertension. *Int J Cardiol* 1998; 64 (2): 179–84.

21 Gonzalez-Juanatey JR, Garcia-Acuna JM, Pose A, Varela A, Calvo C, Cabezas-Cerrato J, de la Pena MG. Reduction of QT and QTc dispersion during long-term treatment of systemic hypertension with enalapril. *Am J Cardiol* 1998; 81 (2): 170–4.

22 Singh JP, Johnston J, Sleight P, Bird R, Ryder K, Hart G. Left ventricular hypertrophy in hypertensive patients is associated with abnormal rate adaptation of QT interval. *J Am Coll Cardiol* 1997; 29 (4): 778–84.

23 Gladman G, Davis AM, Fogelman R, Hamilton RM, Gow RM. TdP, acquired complete heart block and inappropriately long QT in childhood. *Can J Cardiol* 1996; 12 (7): 683–5.

24 Kurita T, Ohe T, Marui N *et al.* Bradycardia-induced abnormal QT prolongation in patients with complete heart block with torsades de pointes. *Am J Cardiol* 1992; 69: 628–33.

25 Kawasaki R, Machado C, Reinoehl J, Fromm B, Baga JJ, Steinman RT, Lehmann MH. Increased propensity of women to develop torsades de pointes during complete heart block. *J Cardiovasc Electrophysiol* 1995; 6 (11): 1032–8.

26 Brachmann J, Scherlag BJ, Rosenshtraukh LV, Lazzara R. Bradycardia-dependent triggered activity: relevance to drug-induced multiform ventricular tachycardia. *Circulation* 1983; 68: 846–56.

27 Shimizu W, Tanaka K, Suenaga K, Wakamoto A. Bradycardia-dependent early afterdepolarizations in a patient with QTU prolongation and torsade de pointes in association with marked bradycardia and hypokalemia. *Pacing Clin Electrophysiol* 1991; 14 (7): 1105–11.

28 Ichida F, Fatica NS, O'Loughlin JE, Snyder MS, Ehlers KH, Engle MA. Correlation of the electrocardiographic and echocardiographic changes in Kawasaki syndrome. *Am Heart J* 1988; 116: 812–9.

29 Ramamurthy S, Talwar KK, Goswami KC, Shrivastava S, Chopra P, Broor S, Malhotra A. Clinical profile of biopsy proven idiopathic myocarditis. *Int J Cardiol* 1991; 41: 225–32.

30 Liberman L, Hordof AJ, Alfayyadh M, Salafia CM, Pass RH. Torsade de pointes in a child with acute rheumatic fever. *J Pediatr* 2001; 138 (2): 280–2.

CHAPTER 11

Acquired long QT syndrome secondary to noncardiac conditions

Diabetes mellitus

Numerous reports have shown that insulin-dependent diabetic patients have a higher incidence of QT prolongation than healthy subjects, particularly those with autonomic neuropathy [1–3]. The prevalence of a QTc interval > 440 ms (Bazett's correction) was reported to be 30.8% in diabetic neuropathic patients, compared with 25.6% in diabetic non-neuropathic patients and 7.6% in healthy controls [3]. TdP has been reported in non insulin-dependent diabetics with QT prolongation [4].

The QT interval significantly correlated with the diabetic autonomic neuropathy score of autonomic cardiovascular test results [5] and both the low and high frequency component of spectral analysis of the R-R interval in diabetic patients, confirming that it is an indicator of cardiac sympathetic and parasympathetic nervous dysfunction [6]. Further study also showed that the QT interval in insulin-dependent diabetic patients was independently associated with age, HbA1c and blood pressure as well as ischemic heart disease and nephropathy [7].

It has been suggested that QT prolongation in diabetic neuropathic patients may be associated with sudden cardiac death in these patients but the evidence for such a link is weak. However, QT prolongation in diabetic patients receiving maintenance hemodialysis was associated with complex ventricular premature complexes (couplets or salvos) and was a predictor of overall mortality in insulin-dependent diabetic nephropathic patients, independent of the presence of autonomic neuropathy [8,9]. Furthermore, in newly diagnosed noninsulin-dependent diabetic patients, maximum the QTc interval is a significant predictor of cardiac mortality [10]. The QT/RR relationships in diabetic patients with autonomic neuropathy are altered, and the changes in the QT interval with time parallel changes in autonomic function [11]. Among the diabetic patients with autonomic neuropathy, the QT interval was significantly longer in those that died (mostly from sudden death), despite similar ages and duration of diabetes. Patients with diabetic autonomic neuropathy had a proportionally greater degree of QT prolongation for a given increase in RR interval, which may at least partly explain the higher incidence of sudden death in these patients [12].

Obesity

While dieting and weight loss on selected diets such as liquid protein diet are associated with prolongation of the QT interval, obesity itself is also a risk factor for repolarization abnormality. There is a correlation between body mass index (BMI) and QT interval, with longer intervals observed in obese subjects [13] although another study did not find any association between obesity and QT prolongation [14]. In premenopausal women, the QT interval is longer in subjects with upper body obesity compared with lower body obesity even at the same level of body fat in moderately obese women. Thus, it is possible that it is only a certain form of obesity (i.e., abdominal obesity) that may prolong ventricular repolarization, at least in premenopausal women [15]. The QT interval correlated closely with plasma free fatty acids and catecholamine concentrations [16] and weight reduction with conventional low calorie diet shortened the QT interval observed in obese patients [17].

Anorexia nervosa

QT prolongation has been observed in patients with anorexia nervosa preceding sudden death [18]. A more recent study reported that patients with anorexia nervosa have a significant increase in baseline QT interval (421 ms, range 334–500 ms) compared with matched controls (390 ms, range 343–444 ms) [19]. In female anorexia nervosa patients, low weight, low body mass index and rapid rate of weight loss immediately preceding the examination were the most important independent predictors of QT interval prolongation despite normal serum potassium, magnesium and calcium levels, indicating that the QT interval is dependent on the degree of "leanness" as well as the prevailing nutritional state (catabolism or anabolism) [20]. The QT interval in anorexia nervosa normalized upon re-feeding, normally within 3 days of re-feeding [21,22]. If a patient with anorexia nervosa develops QT prolongation, the risk of arrhythmia and sudden death must be cautioned. The mechanism of QT prolongation in anorexia nervosa is unknown. Cardiac muscle is lost in proportion to loss of body mass and there is no convincing evidence of impairment of ventricular function in these patients. Abnormalities of the hypothalamus are well described and increased autonomic tone has been suggested as a possible mechanism for lengthening the QT interval [23].

Metabolic causes

Hypokalaemia is by far the commonest metabolic cause of acquired long QT syndrome (Figs 11.1 and 11.2), mainly as a result of diuretic use [24]. Case reports of TdP due to chronic mild hypokalaemia, secondary to diuretic use, hyperaldosteronism and familial periodic paralysis have also been described [25–27]. In the *in-vivo* rat model, hypokalaemia does not affect the delayed

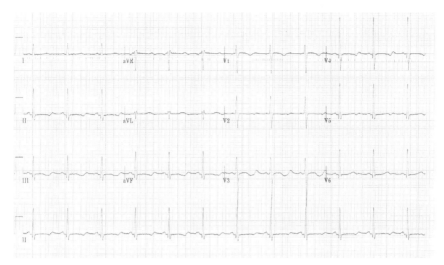

Fig. 11.1 Acquired long QT syndrome in a patient with severe hypokalaemia (2.6 mmol/L). Note the prolonged QT interval of 639 ms and abnormal bizarre T/U wave.

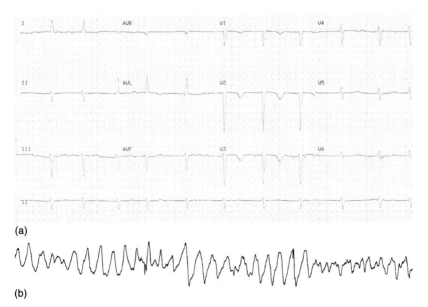

(a)

(b)

Fig. 11.2 An 80-year-old-woman with long-standing unexplained hypokalaemia developed diuretic-induced QT prolongation (QTcB = 705 ms) (a), TdP (b) and cardiac arrest, for which she was resuscitated with D/C cardioversion. Her serum potassium at the time was 3.2 mmol/L after being prescribed coamilofruse despite being on spironolactone and potassium supplementation.

rectifier potassium current, I_{Kr} or the transient outward current, I_{to}. However, hypokalaemia can inhibit the inward rectifier potassium current I_{K1} and thus result in QT prolongation [28].

Other metabolic abnormalities such as hypocalcaemia [29,30] and hypomagnesaemia [31] can also cause QT interval prolongation and may provoke TdP.

Hepatic impairment

As discussed in Chapter 4, drug-induced QT prolongation and TdP were accentuated in patients with hepatic failure [32,33]. Patients with cirrhosis had higher incidence of prolonged QTc interval (>440 ms) compared with controls with mild chronic active hepatitis (46.8% vs. 5.4%, $P < 0.001$) [29]. Another study reported an even higher incidence (83%) of prolonged QTc (>440 ms) in patients with end-stage liver disease [30]. Furthermore, multivariate analysis showed that plasma norepinephrine [34] and Child–Pugh score [34,35] were independently correlated with QTc duration. Thus, in patients with liver cirrhosis, sympathoadrenergic hyperactivity and poor prognostic score represent a risk factor for QT prolongation. However, it is unclear whether QT interval can be used as a prognostic marker of liver dysfunction.

Repolarization abnormalities with prolonged QT intervals and sudden cardiac death have been reported to be associated with chronic alcoholism but the basic arrhythmogenic effect of alcohol is still insufficiently delineated [36,37], although it may be related to sympathoadrenergic hyperactivity.

Intracranial hemorrhage

The electrocardiographic features associated with acute injury of the central nervous system include prominent U waves of either polarity and QT interval prolongation, often exceeding 60% of the normal value, as well as malignant forms of bradycardia and tachycardia. Other electrocardiographic abnormalities include diffuse, deeply inverted T waves [38]. The amplitude of the T wave inversion is marked, approaching 15 mm in some cases. Morphologically, the T wave is asymmetrical with a characteristic outward bulge in the ascending portion. Following an acute cranial injury, relatively minor degrees of ST segment elevation are also seen in leads with abnormal T waves; the ST segment elevation frequently is less noticeable than the T wave changes and is usually less than 3 mm. The T wave inversions with associated ST segment elevation are most pronounced in the midprecordial and lateral precordial leads. Such findings are also noted to a lesser extent in the limb leads.

QT prolongation and TdP were reported to be associated with subarachnoid (Fig. 11.3) and brainstem hemorrhage [39,40]. In a prospective study of

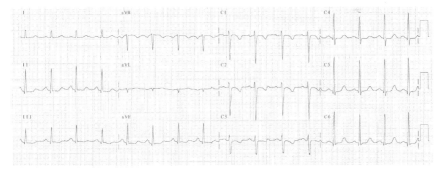

Fig. 11.3 An ECG showing abnormal repolarization with T wave inversion of a middle-age female patient with intracranial hemorrhage.

70 patients with subarachnoid hemorrhage, QT prolongation of $\geq$500 ms was observed in 26% of the patients, with three patients developing TdP within 24 h [39]. QT prolongation, with TU wave alternans and TdP have also been observed to follow brainstem hemorrhage and left thalamus hematoma [40,41]. In a case report of a patient with subarachnoid hemorrhage and drug-refractory TdP, QT prolongation immediately normalized and the arrhythmia was suppressed after left cardiac sympathetic denervation [42]. Thus, sympathetic imbalance has been suggested as the mechanism behind QT prolongation and TdP associated with intracranial hemorrhage [43].

Hypothyroidism

Bradycardia, low voltage ECG (including low voltage P wave, flat or inverted T wave and low R wave), cardiac enlargement and atrio-ventricular block are recognized cardiac complications of hypothyroidism. A well documented but mostly overlooked sign in hypothyroidism is the prolongation of the QT interval. Numerous case reports showed an association between hypothyroidism, QT prolongation, TdP and repeated ventricular fibrillation episodes [44–47]. After thyroid replacement therapy, the QT interval normalized and the patients no longer exhibited any documented arrhythmia [44,45,47]. In one retrospective study of 92 patients with hypothyroidism, the QTc intervals were found to range from 330 to 600 ms (mean 420 ms), but the frequency of QT prolongation or its relationship with the severity of hypothyroidism were not reported [48]. However, another study showed that prolonged QT interval (QTc $\geq$ 450 ms) was only present in 3/14 patients with hypothyroidism (free thyroxin index: 1.5–2.7) and there was no correlation between the degree of QT prolongation and severity of hypothyroidism [46]. The mechanism of hypothyroidism on QT prolongation and the occurrence of ventricular tachycardia is unknown and the effect may be idiosyncratic, although coexistent hypoadrenalism might have contributed to the marked repolarization abnormality [49].

Liquid protein diet

In 1976, following the publication of the book entitled *The Last Chance*, several liquid-protein-modified-fat diets became very popular and fashionable as the dieter's only source of calories and means of rapid weight reduction. Patients taking liquid protein diets had been reported to suffer from syncopal episodes secondary to TdP, ventricular fibrillation and even death after losing a substantial amount of weight. Of note, the use of liquid protein diet can result in hypokalemia, which may predispose the patients to TdP. The ECG's abnormalities include prominent U waves, QT prolongation, ST and T wave abnormalities and left axis deviation [50–53].

Between January 1977 and December 1977, it was estimated that more than 100 000 persons in the US had used one or more of the liquid-protein-modified-fat diets as their sole source of nourishment for at least 1 month. However, between July 1977 and January 1978, at least 60 deaths among avid users of liquid-protein-modified-fat diet were reported to the Food and Drug Administration and Center for Disease Control [54]. In one report, 17 patients died suddenly and unexpectedly during or shortly after using the liquid-protein-modified-fat diet [55]. Sixteen of the 17 patients were female and most were young (mean age 37 years) who lost a substantial amount of weight (mean of 41 kg or 35% of their predicted weight) over a short period of time (mean of 5 months) [55]. Eight patients had one or more episodes of syncope and in the 10 patients that had multilead ECGs recorded; all had ventricular tachycardia and nine patients had QT prolongation (seven had no recognized causes of QT prolongation). Postmortem examination revealed morphological changes on the myocardium, which included attenuated myocardial fibers, increased lipofusin pigment and mononuclear-cell myocarditis. However, these histological changes were not specific and also found in cachetic control subjects, but ECGs in these patients did not show QT prolongation or ventricular tachycardia. Thus the pathogenesis of QT prolongation with liquid protein diets remains unclear. There has been no evidence of toxins in the liquid protein products, especially dioxins, organohalogens, organophosphorous compounds, and the content of heavy metals was below hazardous levels. It has been suggested that it was perhaps starvation itself that produced pathologic alterations of the hypothalamic–pituitary axis of the central nervous system, which precipitated the genesis of ventricular arrhythmias. Other found that ganglionitis and neuritis in the sinus node area and myocarditis induced by liquid protein diet may have predisposed to the QT prolongation and ventricular tachycardia [53].

Physiological variables that prolong the QT interval

Female gender

Female gender deserves special attention as a risk factor for acquired LQTS and TdP, from drug-induced causes. Women are more at risk of developing drug-induced TdP than men [56–58]. A survey on 3135 patients from 22 trials on d,l-sotalol [57] found that TdP was more common in women than men when treated with d,l-sotalol (33/799 vs. 44/2336, $P < 0.001$). The FDA MEDWATCH database showed a female predominance in the drug-associated cardiac arrhythmias including erythromycin, terfenadine, astemizole, halofantrine, quinidine, d-sotalol and other miscellaneous drugs [56,58]. This finding was supported by *in vitro* experiments that erythromycin infusion caused significantly greater QT prolongation in female rabbit hearts than male rabbit hearts (11.8% vs. 6.9%, $P = 0.03$) [56]. Such a difference may be due to the gender difference in specific cardiac ion densities.

In isolated perfused rabbit hearts, the female displayed greater baseline and drug-induced (quinidine and d-sotalol) changes in QT intervals than did male rabbit hearts, and at least two repolarizing potassium current densities (I_{Kr} and I_{K1}) were found to be significantly lower in female cardiomyocytes compared with those from males. Thus, there seems to be clear gender differences in the electrophysiologic characteristics governing cardiac repolarization in animal models [58]. Females are also more susceptible than males to developing TdP in bradycardia-induced LQTS secondary to acquired complete heart block [59]. Thus, women have increased propensity to develop TdP in various settings of QT prolongation.

Age

There is a positive correlation between QTc interval and age, irrespective of the gender [60–62]. The QTc interval increased from $389\pm3\,$ms to $411 \pm 4\,$ms and then to $418 \pm 3\,$ms in patients <30 to 30–65 and >65 years of age [60].

Circadian rhythm

The circadian variability of QT interval is largely responsible for the spontaneous QT variability within individuals. In normal subjects, the diurnal QTc variation ranges from 66 to 95 ms [63–66]. Therefore, any intrasubject variation in QTc interval of less than this range may be regarded as normal and due to circadian variability.

At a given heart rate, the QT interval is longer during sleep than during the awake state [67,68]. The difference in QT interval between awake and sleep states was $19 \pm 7\,$ms when calculated at a heart rate of 60 bpm [67]. Prolongation of the QT interval during sleep may be related to either increased vagal tone or sympathetic withdrawal [67]. However, whether these changes in repolarization at night may explain the diurnal variation of some ventricular arrhythmias remains to be substantiated.

References

1 Bellavere F, Ferri M, Guarini L, Bax G, Piccoli A, Cardone C, Fedele D. Prolonged QT period in diabetic autonomic neuropathy: a possible role in sudden cardiac death. *Br Heart J* 1988; 59: 379–83.

2 Chambers JB, Sampson MJ, Sprigings DC, Jackson G. QT prolongation on the electrocardiogram in diabetic autonomic neuropathy. *Diabet Med* 1990; 7: 105–10.

3 Sivieri R, Veglio M, Chinaglia A, Scaglione P, Cavallo-Perin P. Prevalence of QT prolongation in type 1 diabetic population and its association with autonomic neuropathy. The Neuropathy Study Group of the Italian Society for the Study of Diabetes. *Diabet Medical* 1993, 10, 920–4.

4 Abo K, Ishida Y, Yoshida R *et al.* Torsades de pointes in NIDDM with long QT intervals. *Diabetes Care* 1996; 19 (9): 1010.

5 Veglio M, Chinaglia A, Borra M, Perin PC. Does abnormal QT interval prolongation reflect autonomic dysfunction in diabetes patients? QTc interval measure versus standardized tests in diabetic autonomic neuropathy. *Diabet Med* 1995; 12: 302–6.

6 Oka H, Mochio S, Sato K, Katayama K. Prolongation of the QTc interval and autonomic nervous dysfunction in diabetic patients. *Diabetes Res Clin Pract* 1996; 31: 63–70.

7 Veglio M, Borra M, Stevens LK, Fuller JH, Perin PC. The relation between QTc interval prolongation and diabetic complications. The EURODIAB IDDM Complication Study Group. *Diabetologia* 1999; 42: 68–75.

8 Suzuki R, Tsumura K, Inoue T, Kishimoto H, Morii H. QT interval prolongation in the patients receiving maintenance hemodialysis. *Clin Nephrol* 1998; 49: 240–4.

9 Sawicki PT, Dahne R, Bender R, Berger M. Prolonged QT interval as a predictor of mortality in diabetic nephropathy. *Diabetologia* 1996; 39: 77–81.

10 Naas AAO, Davidson NC, Thompson C *et al.* QT and QTc dispersion are accurate predictors of cardiac death in newly diagnosed noninsulin dependent diabetes: cohort study. *BMJ* 1998; 316: 745–6.

11 Ewing DJ, Boland O, Neilson JM, Cho CG, Clarkes BF. Autonomic neuropathy, QT interval lengthening, and unexpected death in male diabetic patients. *Diabetologia* 1991; 34 (3): 182–5.

12 Bellavere F, Ferri M, Guarini L, Bax G, Piccoli A, Cardone C, Fedele D. Prolonged QT period in diabetic autonomic neuropath: a possible role in sudden cardiac death? *Br Heart J* 1988; 59 (3): 379–83.

13 Pietrobelli A, Rothacker D, Gallagher D, Heymsfield SB. Electrocardiographic QTC interval: short-term weight loss effects. *Int J Obes Relat Metab Disord* 1997; 21: 110–14.

14 Girola A, Enrini R, Garbetta F, Tufano A, Caviezel F. QT dispersion in uncomplicated human obesity. *Obes Res* 2001; 9: 71–7.

15 Park JJ, Swan PD. Effect of obesity and regional adiposity on the QTc interval in women. *Int J Obes Relat Metab Disord* 1997; 21: 1104–10.

16 Corbi GM, Carbone S, Ziccardi P *et al.* FFAs and QT intervals in obese women with visceral adiposity: effects of sustained weight loss over 1 year. *J Clin Endocrinol Metab* 2002; 87: 2080–3.

17 Mshui ME, Saikawa T, Ito K, Hara M, Sakata T. QT interval and QT dispersion before and after diet therapy in patients with simple obesity. *Proc Soc Exp Biol Med* 1999; 220: 133–8.

18 Isner JM, Roberts WC, Heymsfield SB, Yager J. Anorexia nervosa and sudden death. *Ann Intern Med* 1985; 102: 49–52.

19 Durakovic Z, Durakovic A, Korsic M. Changes of the corrected Q-T interval in the electrocardiogram of patients with anorexia nervosa. *Int J Cardiol* 1994; 45: 115–20.

20 Swenne I, Larsson PT. Heart risk associated with weight loss in anorexia nervosa and eating disorders: risk factors for QTc interval prolongation and dispersion. *Acta Paediatr* 1999; 88: 304–9.

21 Cooke RA, Chambers JB, Singh R, Todd GJ, Smeeton NC, Treasure J, Treasure T. QT interval in anorexia nervosa. *Br Heart J* 1994; 72: 69–73.

22 Swenne I. Heart risk associated with weight loss in anorexia nervosa and eating disorders: electrocardiographic changes during the early phase of refeeding. *Acta Paediatr* 2000, 89 (4): 447–52.

23 Thurston J, Marks P. Electrocardiographic abnormalities in patients with anorexia nervosa. *Br Heart J* 1974; 36: 719–23.

24 Takahashi N, Ito M, Inoue T *et al.* Torsades de pointes associated with acquired QT syndrome: observation of 7 cases. *J Cardiol* 1993; 23 (1): 99–106.

25 Chvilicek JP, Hurlbert BJ, Hill GE. Diuretic-induced hypokalaemia inducing torsades de pointes. *Can J Anesth* 1995; 42 (12): 1137–9.

26 Curry P, Fitchett D, Stubbs W, Krikler D. Ventricular arrhythmias and hypokalaemia. *Lancet* 1976; 2: 231–3.

27 Williams MJ, Hammond-Tooke GD, Restieaux NJ. Hypokalaemic periodic paralysis with cardiac arrhythmia and prolonged QT interval. *Aust N Z J Medical* 1995; 25 (5): 549.

28 Hirota M, Ohtani H, Hanada E, Sato H, Kotaki H, Uemura H, Nakaya H, Iga T. Influence of extracellular K+ concentrations on quinidine-induced K+ current inhibition in rat ventricular myocytes. *J Pharm Pharmacol* 2000; 52 (1): 99–105.

29 Akiyama T, Batchelder J, Worsman J, Moses HW, Jedlinski M. Hypocalcemic torsades de pointes. *J Electrocardiol* 1989; 22: 89–92.

30 Davis TM, Singh B, Choo KE, Ibrahim J, Spencr JL, St John A. Dynamic assessment of the electrocardiographic QT interval during citrate infusion in healthy volunteers. *Br Heart J* 1995; 73: 523–6.

31 Kay GN, Plumb VJ, Arciniegas JG, Henthorn RW, Waldo AL. Torsades de pointes: the long-short initiating sequence and other clinical features; observation in 32 patients. *J Am Coll Cardiol* 1983; 2: 806–17.

32 Stanek EJ, Simko RJ, DeNofrio D, Pavri BB. Prolonged quinidine half-life with associated toxicity in a patient with hepatic failure. *Pharmacology* 1997; 17: 622–5.

33 Barre J, Mallat A, Rosenbaum J, Deforges L, Houin G, Dhumeaux D, Tillement JP. Pharmacokinetics of erythromycin in patients with severe cirrhosis. Respective influence of decreased serum binding and impaired liver metabolic capacity. *Br J Clin Pharmacol* 1987; 23: 753–7.

34 Bernardi M, Calandra S, Colantoni A *et al.* Q-T interval prolongation in cirrhosis. prevalence, relationship with severity, etiology of the disease and possible pathogenetic factors. *Hepatology* 1998; 27: 28–34.

35 Mohamed R, Forsey PR, Davies MK, Neuberger JM. Effect of liver transplantation on QT interval prolongation and autonomic dysfunction in end-stage liver disease. *Hepatology* 1996; 23: 1128–34.

36 Kupari M, Koskinen P. Alcohol, cardiac arrhythmias and sudden death. *Novartis Found Symp* 1998; 216: 68–79.

37 Koide T, Ozeki K, Kaihara S, Kato A, Murao S, Kono H. Etiology of QT prolongation and T wave changes in chronic alcoholism. *Jpn Heart J* 1981; 22 (2): 151–66.

38 Perron AD, Brady WJ. Electrocardiographic manifestations of CNS events. *Am J Emerg Med* 2000; 18 (6): 715–20.

39 Andreoli A, Pasquale G, Pinellii G, Grazi P, Tognetti F, Testa C. Subarachnoid hemorrhage frequency and severity of cardiac arrhythmias. *Stroke* 1987; 18: 558–64.

40 Chao CL, Chen WJ, Chung C, Lee YT. Torsades de pointes and T-alternans in a patient with brainstem hemorrhage. *Int J Cardiol* 1995; 51: 199–201.

41 Rotem M, Constantini S, Shir Y, Cotev S. Life-threatening torsades de pointes arrhythmia associated with head injury. *Neurosurgery* 1988; 23: 89–92.

42 Grossman MA. Cardiac arrhythmias in acute central nervous system disease: successful management with stellate ganglion block. *Ann Intern Med* 1976; 136: 203–7.

43 Viskin S. Long QT syndrome and torsades de pointes. *Lancet* 1999; 354: 1625–33.

44 Izumi C, Inoko M, Kitaguchi S, Himura Y, Iga K, General H, Konishi T. Polymorphic ventricular tachycardia in a patient with adrenal insufficiency and hypothyroidism. *Jpn Circ J* 1998; 62 (7): 543–5.

45 Nesher G, Zion MM. Recurrent ventricular tachycardia in hypothyroidism – report of a case and review of the literature. *Cardiology* 1988; 75 (4): 301–6.

46 Kumar A, Bhandari AK, Rahimtoola SH. Torsade de pointes and marked QT prolongation in association with hypothyroidism. *Ann Intern Med* 1987; 106 (5): 712–3.

47 Fredlund BO, Olsson SB. Long QT interval and ventricular tachycardia of "torsade de pointe" type in hypothyroidism. *Acta Med Scand* 1983; 213 (3): 231–5.

48 Douglas AH, Samuel P. Analysis of electrocardiographic patterns in hypothyroid heart disease. *HY State J Med* 1960; 60: 2227–35.

49 Surawicz B, Mangiardi ML. Electrocardiogram in endocrine and metabolic disorders. In: Rios JC, ed. *Clinical Electrocardiographic Correlations*. Philadelphia: FA Davis, 1977: 243.

50 Singh BN, Gaarder TD, Kanegae T, Goldstein M, Montgomerie JZ, Mills H Liquid protein diets and torsade de pointes. *JAMA* 1978; 240 (2): 115–9.

51 Brown JM, Yetter JF, Spicer MJ, Jones JD. Cardiac complications of protein-sparing modified fasting. *JAMA* 1978; 240 (2): 120–2.

52 Michiel RR, Sneider JS, Dickstein RA, Hayman H, Eich RH. Sudden death in a patient on a liquid protein diet. *N Engl J Med* 1978; 298 (18): 1005–7.

53 Siegel RJ, Cabeen WR Jr, Roberts WC. Prolonged QT interval–ventricular tachycardia syndrome from massive rapid weight loss utilizing the liquid-protein-modified-fast diet: sudden death with sinus node ganglionitis and neuritis. *Am Heart J* 1981; 102 (1): 121–2.

54 Gregg MB. Death associated with liquid protein diets. *Morbidity Mortality Weekly Rep* 1977; 26: 383.

55 Isner JM, Sours HE, Paris AL, Ferrans VJ, Roberts WC. Sudden, unexpected death in avid dieters using the liquid-protein-modified-fast diet. Observations in 17 patients and the role of the prolonged QT interval. *Circulation* 1979; 60 (6): 1401–12.

56 Drici M-D, Knollmann BC, Wang W-X, Woosley RL. Cardiac action of erythromycin: influence of female sex. *JAMA* 1998; 280: 1774–6.

57 Lehmann MH, Hardy S, Archibald D, Quart B, MacNeil DJ. Sex difference in risk of torsades de pointes with d,l-sotalol. *Circulation* 1996; 94: 2534–41.

58 Ebert SN, Liu XK, Woosley RL. Female gender as a risk for drug-induced cardiac arrhythmias. evaluation of clinical experimental evidence. *J Womens Health* 1998; 7: 547–57.

59 Kawasaki R, Machado C, Reinoehl J, Fromm B, Baga JJ, Staiman RT, Lehmann MH. Increased propensity of women to develop torsades de pointes during complete heart block. *J Cardiovasc Electrophysiol* 1995; 6: 1032–8.

60 Mangoni AA, Kinirons MT, Swift CG, Jackson SH. Impact of age on QT interval and QT dispersion in healthy subjects: a regression analysis. *Age Ageing* 2003; 32: 326–31.

61 de Bruyne MC, Hoes AW, Kors JA, Hofman A, van Bemmel JH, Grobbee DE. Prolonged QT interval predicts cardiac and all-cause mortality in the elderly. *The Rotterdam Study Eur Heart J* 1999; 20 (4): 278–84.

62 Reardon M, Malik M. QT interval change with age in an overtly healthy older population. *Clin Cardiol* 1996; 19 (12): 949–52.

63 Morganroth J, Brown AM, Critz S, Crumb WJ, Kunze DL, Lacerda AE, Lopez H. Variability of the QTc interval: impact on defining drug effect and low-frequency cardiac event. *Am J Cardiol* 1993; 72 (6): 26B–31B.

64 Morganroth J, Brozovich FV, McDonald JT, Jacobs BA. Variability of the QT measurement in healthy men, with implications for selection of an abnormal QT value to predict drug toxicity an proarrhythmia. *Am J Cardiol* 1991; 67: 774–6.

65 Pratt CM, Ruberg S, Morganroth J *et al.* Dose–response relation between terfenadine (Seldine) and the QTc interval on scalar electgrocardiogram: distinguishing a drug effect from spontaneous variability. *Am Heart J* 1996; 27: 76–83.

66 Molnar J, Zhang F, Weiss J, Ehlert FA, Rosenthal JE. Diurnal pattern of QTc interval: how long is prolonged? Possible relation to circadian triggers of cardiovascular events. *J Am Coll Cardiol* 1996; 27: 76–83.

67 Browne KF, Prystowsky E, Heger JJ, Chilson DA, Zipes DP. Prolongation of the Q-T interval in man during sleep. *Am J Cardiol* 1983; 52 (1): 55–9.

68 Murakawa Y, Yamashita T, Ajiki K, Sezaki K, Omata M. Ostensible day-night difference of QT prolongation during long-term treatment with antiarrhythmic drugs: reappraisal of the law of "regression to the mean". *J Cardiovasc Pharmacol* 1998; 32 (1): 62–5.

CHAPTER 12

Perspective on drug-induced repolarization changes

Regulatory perspective

As stated previously, the awareness of cardiac proarrhythmic toxicity, especially that related to noncardiovascular or cardiovascular nonantiarrhythmic drugs, is rather novel. Sufficient experience does not exist in the interpretation of mild and borderline signals from preclinical and clinical studies. Academic expert consensus is frequently lacking, including a consensus on some of the most essential issues. At the same time, regulatory decisions must be made. It is therefore not surprising that the regulatory agencies have adopted a safe approach and are possibly overcautious. Thus, the regulatory agencies have sometimes been accused of overreacting and of not adopting consistent and coherent approaches to the approval of different compounds. However, it is much easier to be critical of regulatory agencies than to propose a credible alternative. It seems reasonable to anticipate that once further advances in the understanding of the signals of cardiac toxicity have been made, the hurdles of regulatory approval will become more focused and more precisely defined.

Under the present circumstances, there are a number of questions that need to be addressed during the discussions with regulators. Amongst others, the ability of studies/trials to provide data that allow the distinction between drug-induced and natural QT interval prolongation must be addressed. A crossover design is helpful in this setting and should include not only placebo but also negative control arms involving a compound with similar therapeutic efficacy that is known to have no or very little cardiac toxicity. Treatment/placebo effects as well as patient conditioning, known for instance in psychiatric patients but probably present in many others, might be highlighted in this way. Equally importantly, the precision of the assessment needs to be demonstrated. Careful audit and quality control of electrocardiogram measurement is essential. Crossover arms involving a positive control with a drug of known cardiac toxicity may help to demonstrate the power of the study to detect statistically significant QT interval prolongations, but such studies also raise considerable ethical issues. Of course, the crossover design also leads to well-recognized practical problems. The studies take a longer time to organize and complete and potentially suffer from a higher drop-out rate than would a parallel study. Carry-over effects continue to taunt regulators, but in most instances it is easily possible to include sufficient delay between study arms to eliminate this problem. In the QT context the comparability of data and the consequent advantages of data analysis offered by crossover designs generally overwhelm their practical disadvantage. If properly designed and if combined with precise electrocardiogram measurement, the power of crossover studies may be increased allowing far fewer participants to be studied.

Even when a positive signal is found in preclinical investigations and/or clinical phase I/II studies, the regulators might be satisfied that it does not constitute a practical problem if it can be demonstrated that a QT interval prolongation occurs only in situations that are very unlikely to be reproduced in clinical setting. For instance, QT interval prolongation might be found only with dosages that are well above the potential clinical range even when considering slow or modified metabolism. It is true that almost every chemical entity has been used in suicide attempts but if it can be demonstrated that even with doses that might be expected under such circumstances, the QT interval does not prolong very drastically (e.g., <50 ms) while it remains unchanged with lesser doses which are still above the standard clinical range, the issue of cardiac proarrhythmic toxicity might be sidelined.

The fact that no TdP tachycardia was documented during the development and subsequent postmarketing surveillance of a particular drug is not very helpful in establishing the safety of the drug. TdP may masquerade as syncope, fainting, palpitations, ventricular tachycardia or sudden death. These surrogates are very nonspecific and often the true diagnosis remains obscure until the chance recording of an episode of TdP. While with some drugs, the incidence of TdP tachycardia has been reported in more than 1% of treated patients [1–7], the incidence is less than 1 in 100 000 with other drugs that are also considered unsafe. The prescription database of postmarketing surveillance of cisapride involved 36 743 patients treated mainly for gastro-oesophageal reflux and disorders of gastrointestinal motility. The analysis of the database did not show any association between the use of cisapride and serious disorders of cardiac rhythm: with adjustment for clinical history, use of P450 3A4 inhibitors, and use of drugs that prolong the QT interval, the odds ratio for cisapride and cardiac outcomes was 1.0 (95% confidence interval between 0.3 and 3.7) [8]. However, since the launch of cisapride in 1993, over 30 million prescriptions have been written in the USA and 270 adverse events including TdP and 70 fatalities were reported to the FDA between July 1993 and May 1999 [9,10] (that is, one adverse event was reported for more than 111 000 prescriptions and one fatality for approximately every 430 000 prescriptions—on average each patient was prescribed the drug on about three occasions). Hence, the size of clinical studies would have to be truly enormous to claim drug safety on the basis of the absence of TdP tachycardia.

As already discussed, investigations need to be performed not only with the new drug alone but also in combination with compounds that may modify its metabolism or that might contribute to cardiac proarrhythmic toxicity. Since modifications of ion channels may also occur due to a synergy of two or more completely innocent and individually harmless compounds, comprehensive models lead to an endless number of possibilities that might theoretically need investigation. However, the scale of public health problem resulting from such interactions is rather insignificant, although probably not zero (a case of fatal arrhythmia due to intoxication with floor polish has been recorded [11]). It is therefore not surprising that only the cases of established metabolic interactions are being normally investigated.

Some populations might be at an increased risk of proarrhythmic toxicity. This applies to the elderly who frequently receive multiple drugs with the potential for interaction including those which have not been previously appreciated. Similarly, patients with cardiac, renal, hepatic and other predisposing diseases which may increase the risk of abnormal drug elimination and/or modified metabolism have the potential for increased susceptibility to proarrhythmia. Patients with myocardial hypertrophy and/or heart failure, including those without apparent repolarization abnormalities, also constitute a group with increased proarrhythmic danger.

Finally, the results of studies addressing the potential of cardiac proarrhythmic toxicity have to be considered within the overall frame of risk/benefit assessment of a new drug. The outcome of such an assessment depends on the frequency, magnitude and variety of the QT changes observed and on their potential relationship to adverse events detected in the clinical program, on the safety risks presented by the new drug relative to its therapeutic potential, and also on the availability of clinically effective alternatives with a more favorable safety profile. A good example is the withdrawal of terfenadine from the US market after fexofenadine (the effective metabolite of terfenadine) with a much safer profile [12] (despite one report to the contrary [13]) became available. Although halofantrine is blocking the HERG channel [14], results in substantial QT prolongation [15,16] and may well induce TdP and sudden death [17,18], its overall risk/benefit is miniscule in view of its value for the treatment of otherwise resistant malaria. However, since research of new antimalarial drugs continues [16,19], the risk/benefit ratio of halofantrine may need re-evaluating in the future if an equally effective replacement is found with a substantially lower propensity to cardiac proarrhythmic toxicity.

The labeling implications of the risk–benefit assessment for a drug that prolongs QT interval may be considerable. Most frequently, drugs with borderline potential of cardiac toxicity have restrictions imposed and included in its summary of product characteristics (prescribing information). Limitations imposed range from general warnings to contraindications which might be specific or broad in general and which are generally aimed at reducing the exposure of patients who are likely to be more susceptible to the proarrhythmic effects. As with other noncardiac safety concerns, biochemical monitoring may be required. This mostly concerns the levels of serum potassium since hypokalaemia is one of the predisposing factors.

Means and procedures for electrocardiographic monitoring have also been considered and imposed in some cases although it is questionable whether any of these restrictions are practical with noncardiovascular drugs. Some regulators argue that if the judgement of QT interval prolongation and/or T wave morphological changes is left to physicians without special cardiac training, the precision of the assessment is not guaranteed. In practice, physicians frequently rely on automatic QT interval reading provided by commercial electrocardiographs that may be misleading. Similarly, it is questionable whether small noncardiological practices have the capability of recording electrocardiograms with a sufficient degree of technical precision. This is a very relevant consideration with respect to antipsychotic medications, where it is often quite impossible to perform an electrocardiogram, let alone interpret the recording, with sufficient safety and alacrity to provide the urgent treatment that is necessary. Similarly, antimalarial treatment may be urgently needed in circumstances where an ECG recording is quite impossible.

All these regulatory restrictions are only a part of the safety management of a new drug. In clinical reality, whether or not a patient will benefit from detailed prescribing information depends both on the patient and the prescribing physician. The compliance of physicians with prescribing restrictions and monitoring requirements is poor. In published surveys on terfenadine and cisapride, there was a significant number of inappropriate prescriptions of these drugs to patients at increased risk [20–22]. Monitoring requirements such as baseline and/or periodic ECGs have been frequently ignored. These realizations have made regulatory agencies aware of the fact that prescribing restrictions might not offer the safety net for which they are intended. Some agencies therefore argue that rather than relying on complex and significant prescribing restrictions of a drug is not otherwise essential, it is better not to approve the new compound at all.

Other parts of the safety management of a new drug include patient information sheets and booklets, pharmacy training, healthcare lectures, etc. All these may help until the cardiac safety of a new drug is verified through substantial exposure. It is essential to counsel patients about any risk they face when accepting pharmaceutical therapy. It is our practice to provide all patients at proarrhythmic risk from drug induced QT prolongation an information leaflet, which they are encouraged to read, and show to their doctors, pharmacists and friends. Some websites are freely accessible on the internet for checking out proarrhythmic drugs that prolong QT interval and cause TdP, e.g., http://www.qtdrugs.org.

Academic perspective

Presently, despite numerous attempts [23–32], no automatic method for QT interval measurement as incorporated in existing commercial equipment is reliable enough to be used in studies of drug-induced QT interval prolongation. Even with technologies supplied by leading manufacturers of electrocardiographic equipment, substantial discrepancies appear between automatic and manual measurement by a trained cardiologist [33]. Thus, the most immediate challenge to academia is the development of more advanced automatic measurement techniques. While the simple graphics manipulations of T wave patterns, e.g., various threshold and tangent methods, seem to be remote from the target, some of the new theoretical concepts [34,35] may offer a hope that the problem will not take very long to solve.

The duration of the QT interval is only one of the possible measures of cardiac repolarization. At times when electrocardiograms were solely recorded on paper, other measures such as areas under the T wave in different ECG leads were not practical. At present, however, electrocardiograms are recorded mostly digitally and the digital signals can be easily subjected to complex computer processing. A consensus is now emerging that abnormalities of the morphology of the T wave, which are normally hidden within the clinical diagnosis of "nonspecific T wave changes", are potentially more important than the length of the QT interval. Indeed, the cases of gross QT interval prolongation by drugs with known cardiac toxicity are mostly accompanied by substantial modifications of T wave morphology which is perhaps less easy to miss than the changes of the QT interval duration and which, pending the development of appropriate technology, might be detected with a substantially better accuracy. Academia is therefore facing a substantial challenge of developing both appropriate technical tools for T wave morphology assessment as well relevant physiologic and pathophysiologic models in order to understand the meaning of the new repolarization characteristics. Early indications show that morphological assessment of the T wave is likely to be more potent than the sole measurement of the QT interval [36,37]. It can be expected that this stream of research will have substantial implications for the assessment of cardiac proarrhythmic toxicity and of drug-induced repolarization abnormalities. The measurement of the QT interval is not particularly precise and the association of a prolonged QT interval with proarrhythmic effects is not direct. Therefore, it is likely that in the future, the measurement of the interval will no longer be used for the assessment of drug safety. The morphological descriptors have a potential for not only detecting subtle warnings of cardiac toxicity but also of classifying patients to those more or less susceptible to adverse proarrhythmic effects [38].

The detection and classification of individual susceptibility in addition to the detection of proarrhythmic danger of a new compound is another academic challenge. It is now generally accepted that patients who develop TdP tachycardia on a proarrhythmic drug are those who have a special predisposition to such an adverse reaction. Such a tendency is likely to be multifactorial including genetic predisposition [39,40] such as nonpenetrating penetrant gene abnormality of the congenital long QT interval syndrome or other gene abnormality of cardiac ion channels [41,42]. In this sense, the differences between less or more cardiac toxic drugs might be related to the degree of predisposing abnormality required for proarrhythmia manifestation. Hence, a complete spectrum might exist between cardiac toxicity which manifests by triggering TdP tachycardia even in subjects with a very mild repolarization abnormality and cases of cardiac toxicity with which a rare gene abnormality or other combinations of predisposing factors are more to blame than the drug itself. It seems plausible to speculate that electrocardiographic testing, perhaps combined with special electrophysiologic (e.g., pacing induced long-short-long sequences) or other challenges [43], might be capable of detecting different spectra of diminished repolarization safety-net thus identifying patients in whom the cardiac toxicity of a particular compound is more likely to manifest. If successful, detection of nonpenetrant gene abnormalities might offer the advantage of classifying cardiac safety for individual patients rather than for the general population.

Practical perspective

In clinical practice, adverse effects of QT prolongation secondary to drugs can be prevented by not exceeding the recommended dose, avoiding their use or restricting the dose in patients with pre-existing heart disease or risk factors or other acquired long QT syndrome, previous ventricular arrhythmias and/ or electrolyte imbalance such as hypokalaemia. Concomitant administration of drugs that inhibit the cytochrome P450 3A4 (e.g., imidazole antifungals, macrolide antibiotics) or those that can prolong the QT interval or drugs that cause hypokalaemia should be avoided.

The management of patients with TdP secondary to acquired LQTS includes identifying the cause, replenishing the potassium level to 4.5–5 mmol/L and infusing 1–2 g of bolus of intravenous magnesium over 2–3 min, repeated if necessary, and followed by an infusion of 2–8 mg/min. If the TdP is drug-induced, the offending drug(s) should be withdrawn. In resistant cases, temporary cardiac pacing at a rate of 90/min or isoproterenol may be needed to increase the heart rate and shorten the QT interval. Isoproterenol, however, should only be used if: (i) the cardiac pacing cannot be started immediately; (ii) there is an underlying bradycardia; and (iii) TdP is pause-dependent. Intravenous beta-blockers have a role in the management of "arrhythmia storms" not responsive to magnesium, if the underlying rhythm is sinus tachycardia, or if the patient is protected from excessive pause by cardiac pacing.

References

1 Selzer A, Wray HW. Quinidine syncope. Paroxysmal ventricular fibrillation occurring during treatment of chronic atrial arrhythmias. *Circulation* 1964; 30: 17–26.
2 Roden DM, Woosley RL, Primm RK. Incidence and clinical features of the quinidine–associated long QT syndrome: implications for patient care. *Am Heart J* 1986; 111: 1088–93.

3 Kay GN, Plumb VJ, Arciniegas JG *et al.* Torsade de pointes: the long-short initiating sequence and other clinical features: observations in 32 patients. *J Am Coll Cardiol* 1983; 2: 806–17.

4 Bauman JL, Bauernfeind RA, Hoff JV *et al.* Torsades de pointes due to quinidine: observations in 31 patients. *Am Heart J* 1984; 107: 425–30.

5 Haverkamp W, Martinez RA, Hief C *et al.* Efficacy and safety of d,l-sotalol in patients with ventricular tachycardia and in survivors of cardiac arrest. *J Am Coll Cardiol* 1997; 30: 487–95.

6 Lehmann MH, Hardy S, Archibald D *et al.* Sex difference in risk of torsade de pointes with d,l-sotalol. *Circulation* 1996; 94: 2535–41.

7 Hohnloser SH. Proarrhythmia with class III antiarrhythmic drugs: types, risks and management. *Am J Cardiol* 1997; 80: 82G–89G.

8 Walker AM, Szeneke P, Weartherby LB *et al.* The risk of serious cardiac arrhythmias among cisapride users in the United Kingdom and Canada. *Am J Med* 1999; 107: 356–62.

9 Food and Drug Administration. Cisapride. *The Pink Sheet*, 31st January 2000.

10 Miller JL. FDA, Janssen bolster cardiac risk warnings for cisapride. *Am J Health Syst Pharm* 2000; 57: 414.

11 Raikhin-Eisenkraft B, Nutenko I, Kniznik D *et al.* Death from fluoro-silicate in floor polish [in Hebrew]. *Harefuah* 1994; 126: 258–9.

12 Pratt C, Brow AM, Rampe D *et al.* Cardiovascular safety of fexofenadine HCl. *Clin Exp Allergy* 1999; 29 (Supl 3): 212–6.

13 Pinto YM, van Gelder IC, Heeringa M *et al.* QT lengthening and life-threatening arrhythmias associated with fexofenadine. *Lancet* 1999; 353: 980.

14 Tie H, Walker BD, Singleton CB *et al.* Inhibition of HERG potasium channels by the antimalarial agent halofantrine. *Br J Pharmacol* 2000; 130: 1967–75.

15 Monlun E, Pillet O, Cochard JF *et al.* Prolonged QT interval with halofantrine. *Lancet* 1993; 341: 1541–2.

16 Wesche DL, Schuster BG, Wang WX *et al.* Mechanism of cardiotoxicity of halofantrine. *Clin Pharmacol Ther* 2000; 67: 521–9.

17 Toivonen L, Viitasalo M, Siikamaki H *et al.* Provocation of ventricular tachycardia by antimalarial drug halofantrine in congenital long QT syndrome. *Clin Cardiol* 1994; 17: 403–4.

18 Akhtar T, Imran M. Sudden deaths while on halofantrine treatments – a report of two cases from peshawar. *JPMA J Pak Med Assoc* 1994; 44: 120–1.

19 Bakshi R, Hermeling-Fritz I, Gathmann I *et al.* An integrated assessment of the clinical safety of artemether-lumefantrine: a new oral fixed-dose combination antimalarial drug. *Trans R Soc Trop Med Hyg* 2000; 94: 419–24.

20 Cavuto NJ, Woosley RL, Sale M *et al.* Pharmacies and prevention of potentially fatal drug interactions. *JAMA* 1996; 275: 1086–7.

21 Thompson D, Oster G. Use of terfenadine and contraindicated drugs. *JAMA* 1996; 275: 1339–41.

22 Janssen propulsid prescribing for inpatients questioned in three studies. *FDC Report "The Pink Sheet"*. 1998; 60: 26.

23 Puddu PE, Bernard PM, Chaitman BR *et al.* QT interval measurement by a computer assisted program: a potentially useful clinical parameter. *J Electrocardiol* 1982; 15: 15–21.

24 Fayn J, Rubel P, Mohsen N. An improved method for the precise measurement of serial ECG changes in QRS duration and QT interval. Performance assessment on the CSE noise-testing database and a healthy 720 case-set population. *J Electrocardiol* 1992; 24 (Suppl.): 123–7.

25 Bhullar HK, Fothergill JC, Goddard WP *et al*. Automated measurement of QT interval dispersion from hard-copy ECGs. *J Electrocardiol* 1993; 26: 321–31.

26 Laguna P, Jane R, Caminal P. Automatic detection of wave boundaries in multilead ECG signals: validation with the CSE database. *Comput Biomed Res* 1994; 27: 45–60.

27 Rubel P, Hamidi S, Behlouli H *et al*. Are serial Holter QT, late potential, and wavelet measurement clinically useful? *J Electrocardiol* 1996; 29 (Suppl.): 52–61.

28 Reddy BR, Xue Q, Zywietz C. Analysis of interval measurements on CSE multilead reference ECGs. *J Electrocardiol* 1996; 29 (Suppl.): 62–6.

29 Hoon TJ. Performance of an electrocardiographic analysis system: implications for pharmacodynamic studies. *Pharmacotherapy* 1996; 16: 230–6.

30 Glancy JM, Weston PJ, Bhullar HK *et al*. Reproducibility and automatic measurement of QT dispersion. *Eur Heart J* 1996; 17: 1035–9.

31 Xue Q, Reddy S. Algorithms for computerized QT analysis. *J Electrocardiol* 1998; 30: 181–6.

32 Tikkanen PE, Sellin LC, Kinnunen HO *et al*. Using simulated noise to define optimal QT intervals for computer analysis of ambulatory ECG. *Med Eng Phys* 1999; 21: 15–25.

33 Savelieva I, Yi G, Guo X *et al*. Agreement and reproducibility of automatic versus manual measurement of QT interval and QT dispersion. *Am J Cardiol* 1998; 81: 471–7.

34 Vila JA, Yi G, Rodríguez Presedo AM *et al*. A new approach for TU complex characterization. *IEEE Trans Biomed Eng* 2000; 47: 764–72.

35 Acar B, Yi G, Hnatkova K *et al*. Spatial, temporal and wavefront direction characteristics of 12-lead T wave morphology. *Med Biol Eng Comput* 1999; 37: 574–84.

36 Zabel M, Acar B, Klingenheben T *et al*. Analysis of twelve-lead T wave morphology for risk stratification after myocardial infarction. *Circulation* 2000; 102: 1252–7.

37 Hnatkova K, Ryan SJ, Bathen J *et al*. T-wave morphology differentiates between patients with and without arrhythmic complications of ischaemic heart disease. *J Electrocardiol* 2001; 34(Suppl.): 113–17.

38 Zhang L, Timothy KW, Vincent M *et al*. Spectrum of ST-T-wave pattrns and repolarization paramaters in congenital long–QT syndrome: ECG findings identify genotypes. *Circulation* 2000; 102: 2849–55.

39 Sesti F, Abbott GW, Wei J *et al*. A common polymorphism associated with antibiotic-induced cardiac arrhythmia. *Proc Natl Acad Sci* 2000; 97: 10613–8.

40 Napolitano C, Schwartz PJ, Brown AM *et al*. Evidence for a cardiac ion channel mutation underlying drug-induced QT prolongation and life-threatening arrhythmias. *J Cardiovasc Electrophysiol* 2000; 11: 691–6.

41 Clancy CE, Rudy Y. Linking a genetic defect to its cellular phenotype in a cardiac arrhythmia. *Nature* 1999; 400: 566–9.

42 Roden DM, Kupershmidt S. From genes to channels: normal mechanisms. *Cardiovasc Res* 1999; 42: 318–26.

43 Darbar D, Smith M, Morike K *et al*. Epinephrine-induced changes in serum potassium and cardiac repolarization and effects of pretreatment with propranolol and diltiazem. *Am J Cardiol* 1996; 77: 1351–5.

Index